T0031086

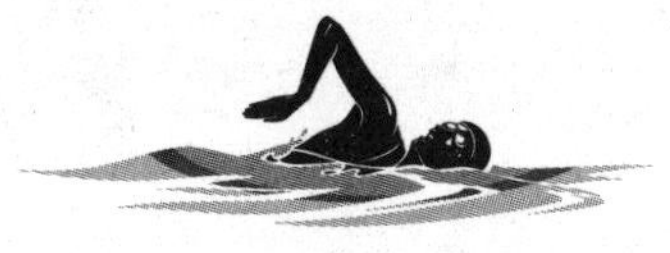

Chill

A TRANSFORMATIVE GUIDE TO RENEW YOUR BODY & MIND

Chill

THE COLD WATER SWIM CURE

MARK HARPER, MD, PhD

CHRONICLE PRISM

Library of Congress Cataloging-in-Publication Data
Names: Harper, Mark (Anaesthetist), author.
Title: Chill : the cold water swim cure / Mark Harper, MD, PHD.
Description: 1st. | San Francisco : Chronicle Prism, [2022] | "A transformative guide to renew your body and mind"—Cover. | Includes bibliographical references. |
Identifiers: LCCN 2022004208 (print) | LCCN 2022004209 (ebook) | ISBN 9781797213767 (paperback) | ISBN 9781797213781 (ebook)
Subjects: LCSH: Swimming—Therapeutic use. | Swimming—Physiological aspects.
Classification: LCC RC1220.S8 H37 2022 (print) | LCC RC1220.S8 (ebook) | DDC 613.7/16—dc23/eng/20220217
LC record available at https://lccn.loc.gov/2022004208
LC ebook record available at https://lccn.loc.gov/2022004209

Manufactured in the United States of America.

Design by Brooke Johnson. Typesetting by Maureen Forys, Happenstance Type-O-Rama. Typeset in Atlantik, Filosofia, Gotham, Knockout, Karmina, and Sackers Gothic.

10 9 8 7 6 5 4 3 2 1

CHRONICLE PRISM

Chronicle Prism is an imprint of Chronicle Books LLC, 680 Second Street, San Francisco, California 94107
www.chronicleprism.com

Contents

PART II
THE COLD WATER SWIM PROTOCOL

PART III
THE COLD WATER SWIM CURE

Author's Note

In 1760, more than two centuries before I first dipped my toes in the frigid waters off Brighton, Dr. Richard Russell, a renowned physician, published his famous "Dissertation on the use of sea water in the diseases of the glands: Particularly the scurvy, jaundice, King's-evil, leprosy, and the glandular consumption."

As part of his prescription, Dr. Russell recommended patients regularly swim in the ocean and, postswim, drink pints of seawater mixed with "an oxymel of squills," an effective purgative.

While most of Dr. Russell's claims may be somewhat overambitious—and, admittedly, rather unpalatable—I have no doubt he observed in his research and his treatment regimens real positive effects.

I have witnessed similar effects.

Since Dr. Russell's prime, our knowledge of physiology has advanced considerably. We can now explain, for instance, his observations about swimming in open water, particularly in water below 68°F, or 20°C. We also know more about what happens to the body when it is exposed to cold water, how the body adapts to the stress of cold water over time, and how regular cold water swimming can help people cope with the ill effects of modern life—from chronic pain and osteoarthritis to migraines, depression, and anxiety.

Of course, I don't suggest that sea bathing has all the benefits Dr. Russell described. Nor do I recommend following his radical regime of bloodletting and ingesting seawater alongside a tincture of ipecacuanha (an emetic), carduus water, squill, spodium, raw egg yolk with the "fome" of the white, cinnamon, and sugar candy. To be honest, I can't promise that cold water swimming is a definitive cure for any particular symptom or ailment, no matter how many hours someone logs in the water. Unlike Dr. Russell, I do not believe swimming in cold water alone is some kind of universal cure.

That said, scientific evidence and first-person accounts show that cold water swimming is an effective therapeutic when practiced with other forms of medical interventions and consistent changes in lifestyle habits for which it may be the catalyst.

I provide that evidence and those stories in the following pages, which clearly demonstrate the very real, life-changing health effects of regular dips in temperate to frigid waters. The reason for this is that cold water swimming combines a number of the best and most effective aspects of preventative medicine and, more importantly, healthy living. Cold water swimming results in immediate—and sustainable—improvements in overall health and general well-being across three essential categories: reorientation, transformation, and connection.

Cold water swimmers report an overall improvement in both their physical and mental health. This includes reductions in blood pressure, inflammation, and chronic pain levels, as well as weight loss, better sleep, and a more engaged and optimistic outlook. There are additional knock-on benefits that include greater resilience and a more substantial place within the community, which reduces social isolation and provides a shared sense of caring and belonging. Cold water swimming enhances personal autonomy, encourages personal achievement, and is an opportunity to spend time outdoors, which in itself improves our overall well-being.

Plus, importantly, it's fun. All of this provides a significant boost to our system and lets us reboot our body and mind, which is the first step to feeling revitalized and refreshed and consequently enjoying a healthier and more satisfying life.

I have divided the book into three parts. In part I, "The Transformative Power of Water," I explain in everyday language how cold water swimming improves general well-being—including the science of cold water immersion and cold water adaptation. In part II, "The Cold Water Swim Protocol," I provide advice for cold water swimming itself. This includes making a plan, finding companions, and having the proper kit, but most of all, how to do it: getting in and getting out, getting wet and getting blessedly dry and warm. In part III, "The Cold Water Swim Cure," I provide inspiring first-person accounts of how a consistent cold water swimming practice has improved the symptoms of a range of mental and physical illnesses, such as depression and trauma, chronic pain, migraines, fibromyalgia, and autoimmune diseases.

Now, if you're ready to take the plunge, let's dive in.

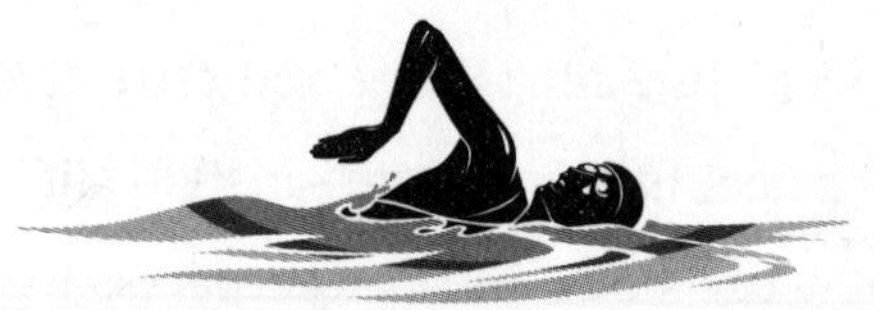

PART I

The Transformative Power of Water

CHAPTER 1

THAT'S FUNNY

My Cold Water Epiphanies

I'VE ALWAYS SWUM.

For several summers as a young man, I worked as a lifeguard on the beaches of Brighton. Fortunately, the swimmers I was charged with protecting rarely got into real difficulty. In fact, I never once had to venture into the surf, largely because back in the 1980s neither I nor many of my fellow countrymen and -women seemed to have any inclination to set foot in the cold water.

As I grew older and progressed through my career in medicine, I continued to train in the swimming pools of London. After finishing my postgraduate training in anesthesia, I returned to Brighton for a consultant post in 2003, which is when I started training with Brighton Swimming Club, the oldest such club in

England. Happily, I took full advantage of their heated pool, which was open all year, save for two weeks every summer. After hearing me moan about this minor inconvenience, my old friend Jasper suggested I join the club's sea-swimming group that swam in the English Channel—to my considerable surprise—year-round, regardless of the temperature.

Confident in my abilities, and not in the slightest bit worried about being out of my literal and figurative depths, I was nevertheless apprehensive about swimming in the cold water. I was accustomed to swimming in heated pools, and I knew how cold the sea was, having regularly participated, somewhat reluctantly, in the club's annual Pier-to-Pier race.

Nonetheless, one morning in August 2004, I joined a dozen or so compatriots and steeled myself for what I knew was coming.

The gloriously evocative lines in Iris Murdoch's novel *The Sea* came to my mind as I approached the water's edge: "Trembling with emotion, I tore my clothes off and walked into the sea. The cold shock, then the warmth, then the strong gentle lifting motion of the quiet waves reminded me of happiness."

Fortunately, I didn't need to tear off my clothes—we had a rather grim but effective changing room—but the progression of emotions and sensations Murdoch describes were spot-on.

First—before I could enjoy the strong, gentle, lifting motion of the quiet waves, let alone the warmth or happiness—I had to endure the very real shock of the cold. There's no way around it. Getting into cold water is a shock and a stress. Rather than a detriment, however, although I didn't realize it at the time, this immediate sensation and deeply felt physiological effect is exactly why cold water swimming and other forms of cold immersion therapies are so incredibly effective in reducing symptoms and complications of chronic and acute physical and mental conditions.

Stepping into cold water, you feel the cold engulf every inch of your body, from the soles of your feet to the tip of your nose. At water temperatures of 68°F, or 20°C, the skin vasoconstricts maximally, which is a fancy way of saying the blood vessels that run in our skin completely shut down to insulate the body from the cold. At the same time, stepping into cold water accelerates our heart rate and raises our blood pressure, thanks to the secretion of adrenaline and noradrenaline into our bloodstream.

Cold water also has a dramatic effect on breathing in those not used to it. First, it stimulates a large, involuntary "inspiratory gasp." Anyone who has jumped into cold water, whether by accident or on purpose, has experienced the sharp inhale of breath that occurs reflexively upon submersion. This gasp is followed by rapid breathing, or hyperventilation, which is impossible to override, even for swimmers who are steeled for it.

The consequent stretching of the heart chambers—notably the atria—results in the release of a hormone called "atrial natriuretic peptide." In simple terms, this tells the kidneys to offload more water, which fills the bladder and leaves cold water swimmers with the slightly uncomfortable need to urinate.

As hard as it is to believe, all of this stress can be good for you.

THAT'S FUNNY

While I had swum in the sea before, it had always been as a race or messing around with friends. This was the first occasion I had done so with any kind of consciousness of my body's sensations and of my immediate environment. Since then, I've always thought of this as the first swim of my outdoor swimming "career."

As I emerged from the water, I remembered the words of another writer, Isaac Asimov, who observed, "The most exciting phrase in science isn't 'Eureka,' but 'that's funny.'" I was aware of a number of different sensations: My fingertips were numb, and I had a suspicious lack of strength in my hands and a reduced sensation of feeling all over my body. My feet were also somewhat uncomfortable from walking over the beach's uneven pebbles. Yet, I clearly remember thinking, Hmm. That's funny. I feel really good.

This made me curious about how cold water could have a positive effect on the human body. The body's primary aim is to keep the vital organs—the body's "core"—in the very narrow temperature range of 97.7 to 99.5°F (36.5 to 37.5°C). When the external environment is cool and the body's not generating heat through movement, it shuts down the blood supply to the body's "periphery"—the skin and (inactive) muscles, which become relatively cold in order to insulate the core and keep it warm.

When surgery patients are under anesthesia, however, this insulation system breaks down because anesthetics block the parts of the nervous system that help regulate body temperature. This causes the core to become hypothermic, or too cold, and the body's vital organs stop functioning at an optimal level. This is hardly great under normal circumstances, but following the stress of surgery, it can have serious consequences. This is why anesthetists like me use specially designed hot-air blankets to warm patients throughout their operation.

However, as I read more about the physiological response to cold water immersion, it kept reminding me of the body's physiological response to surgery. This makes sense because both are evolutionary stress responses. As such, the body reacts to these challenges in the same way it reacts to any other kind of stress, whether we're going under the knife, getting chased by a saber-toothed tiger, or running late for an important appointment.

While this stress response has evolved to protect and heal us, following surgery it overreacts, which can exacerbate the adverse effects of hypothermia. This led me to wonder if, by teaching the body how to adapt to the stress of the cold through cold water swimming, it would be possible to reduce the stress reaction in patients undergoing surgery to a "physiological" rather than "pathological" level—and thereby reduce the risk of complications. The more often the body is exposed to cold temperatures, the less intensely the body responds to this exposure and stress as life-threatening.

This was how my initial "that's funny" moment became a working theory about a therapeutic intervention. If patients went through a cold water adaptation program before their operations, I hypothesized, they could lessen the magnitude of the stress response on their bodies, which would maximize and accelerate their recovery. In 2012, I published a paper suggesting this theory in *Medical Hypotheses* entitled "Extreme Preconditioning: Cold Adaptation Through Sea Swimming as a Means to Improving Surgical Outcomes."

The longer I considered this theory, however, the more keenly I suspected cold water adaptation could produce similar mental and physical health benefits far outside of the operating room. Wedding my professional expertise to my newfound passion, I started to study—and practice—cold water swimming in the hope of developing a therapeutic intervention for many of today's most prevalent chronic ailments and conditions.

A (BRIEF) HISTORY OF COLD WATER THERAPIES

I am certainly not the first to champion the positive effects of cold water on our mental and physical health. Nor, indeed, was Dr. Richard Russell. Historically, water has always been considered fundamental to our health and well-being—mentally, physically, and spiritually. Hippocrates, who is commonly thought of as the "father of Western medicine," believed water therapy allayed lassitude, discussing this and more in his treatise "On Air, Waters, and Places."

The ancient Greeks placed great faith in the healing powers of the ocean and the marine environment. Plato claimed the ocean could cure all ailments, while Euripides proclaimed that "the sea washes away all men's illnesses." Hippocrates, Plato, and

Aristotle—they all recommended hot seawater baths because, in Greek medicine, water was believed to have an "expulsive virtue" that washes waste and impurities from the body. With their dips into the frigidarium, the Romans got even closer to the "cold water cure." Cato the Elder, for one, served his slaves a mixture of wine and seawater to restore their depleted energies. Centuries later, Thomas Jefferson soaked his feet in a cold bath every morning to "maintain his good health."

But the importance of water extends beyond Western medical traditions. It has a significant role in many religions: Christianity, Buddhism, Islam, Judaism, and Hinduism. Sacred springs and water deities can be found throughout the world and throughout history.

Perhaps this is why a Greek physician living over two millennia ago and a doctor from my own hometown 250 years ago were really on to something when they celebrated the holistic benefits of water. Ocean bathing reached a peak in popularity in the late eighteenth century around the time of the development of the swimsuit. Whole communities were founded on the perceived health benefits of sea swimming. Brighton itself went from being a sleepy fishing town to the favored resort of the Prince Regent—later George IV—and his court. Since most people didn't know how to swim, women were taken into the water by "dippers," who used "bathing machines" to help them in and out of the water. In a way, these dippers were the forerunners of today's lifeguards. The most famous dipper was a woman named Martha Gunn.

Martha was well-regarded by both the local community and the Prince Regent. She was even entrusted to "dip" his little daughter, Princess Charlotte. I swim with one of Gunn's descendants, Paul Smith, who, rather appropriately, runs a swimming school that teaches people to swim in the ocean and that trains more lifeguards than almost any other single center in the United Kingdom.

Even ten years ago, my practice of year-round ocean bathing was considered eccentric. However, over the last few years, the growth in cold water swimming has been significant, including both competitions—like ice swimming, marathon swimming, winter swimming, and triathlons—and general "wild swimming."

With increased participation has come renewed and enthusiastic claims for the physiological and psychological health benefits of cold water swimming. Winter swimmers claim to have fewer infections than nonswimmers, though the evidence for this remains weak. When combined with breathing techniques, adaptation to cold water seems to modify the body's immune response to an endotoxin challenge, but the clinical implications of this are as yet not clear.

That said, cold water swimming has the potential to alleviate the symptoms of a wide range of conditions—although perhaps not all the "diseases of the glands," as Russell claimed. There is no doubt that it produces a tremendous feeling of energy and wellbeing. I have been ocean swimming for seventeen winters, and I still do not find getting into sub-50°F (sub-10°C) water a pleasant experience. However, I have become addicted to the resultant "euphoria" and the undeniable sense of rejuvenation and unwavering vigor, the duration and magnitude of which seems inversely proportional to the water temperature. Russell wrote about a similar effect on morose boys:

> I have often had boys brought to me, weak and pale, with long thick hair hanging down their necks, and covered up with the greatest care, lest the tender creatures should be killed with the cold, the whole texture of the body being relaxed with the heat of their clothing, and with nocturnal sweats. I have sent them back to their parents, with their hair cut off, their necks bare, with a florid, youthful countenance, having first strengthened their limbs by bathing in the sea.

I know this to be true for myself and anecdotally for others. I know how good I feel after swimming in cold water. And this is what led me to wonder if cold water swimming could also be an effective treatment for depression.

SARAH, THE BBC, AND COLD WATER THERAPY

Interestingly, many of the studies I read about the physiology of cold adaptation came from Professor Mike Tipton and his team in Portsmouth, about fifty miles east of Brighton. An accomplished and prolific researcher, Mike is editor-in-chief of the Physiological Society's journal *Experimental Physiology* and a fellow of both the Royal Society of Medicine and the Physiological Society. For his contribution to physiological research in extreme environments, he was awarded an MBE by the Queen of England, one of the five classes of appointment of the British Empire. Mike literally wrote the book about the physiology of cold water adaptation.

In 2013, Mike and I met while I was helping a friend do research into the effects of cold water swimming on the immune system. I told Mike how his research greatly informed my *Medical Hypotheses* paper, and I explained my theory that cold water adaptation might help treat depression.

Not long after this conversation, Mike was contacted by Chris van Tulleken, a famous TV doctor in England who is basically the UK's Dr. Oz. Chris was looking for ideas for a new documentary series called *The Doctor Who Gave Up Drugs*. Mike told Chris about my theory, and Chris decided to film a segment for the first episode in which somebody who struggles with depression tries cold water swimming for the first time as an alternative to medication.

Diagnosed with depression at the age of fifteen, Sarah had spent nearly a decade on and off antidepressants, including Prozac and Citalopram, which helped but eventually left her feeling emotionally numb. Desperate for her infant daughter, Evie, not to grow up seeing her mom taking pills, Sarah responded to an advertisement she saw in her doctor's office and volunteered for Chris's television program.

"On my worst days, I just wanted to sit in a dark room," she says in the episode. "I managed to keep working but that was about it. I avoided all socializing."

After her father's suicide, she plunged into an even deeper depression, and her doctor prescribed a higher dosage. Then she stopped taking the pills when she became pregnant, and for the first time in years, she felt happy and optimistic—until six months after her daughter's birth, when her brother died from an overdose. "The old feelings returned," she says, "and I was back on Citalopram."

The plan was to start in Mike's specially designed "endless" swimming pool at the University of Portsmouth. She and Chris would do four to six static swims (that is, swimming in place against a manufactured current) over the course of one day—warming up completely in between swims—so she would become adapted to the cold. The following day, she would swim in a nearby lake for her first cold water swim outdoors, in the "wild."

Quite understandably, Sarah found getting into the cold water in Mike's pool very challenging. After her second swim, she almost gave up. "The water was so cold," Sarah says. "I started hyperventilating. It was very emotional, and I broke down after the second immersion." Sarah was, however, highly motivated to get off her medications, and ultimately she managed four immersions that first day. By her third swim, she really started to enjoy being in the cold water.

The next morning, Chris brought Sarah to the lake, where Heather—a senior member of Mike's research team—and I joined them for support. As we stood waist deep in the lake, I could feel how nervous and reluctant Sarah was. "Think of Evie,"

I told her. With that, she let herself go and took to it like, well, a fish to water. Immediately, her pride and courage returned, and she completely overcame her fear. Swimming outside in cold water, surrounded by nature, filled her with joy. The four of us swam laps together. After about four, I was feeling the cold, but Sarah wanted to keep going. When she finally got out, she was a bundle of bubbliness and smiles. "Within a minute or two," she says, "I felt calmer and ended up swimming for twenty minutes. I didn't want to come out. I felt on top of the world afterward. I was hooked."

Following this experience, Sarah continued with a lake swim once a week and even started taking cold baths at home. Over the next few months, she tapered down her Citalopram and, eventually, got off all her medications.

"I still have my ups and downs," she says, "but I deal with them by swimming. It's changed my attitude to everything. I've been to toddler groups with Evie—something I couldn't have contemplated before. Swimming and socializing have helped me more than pills ever did."

The BBC program aired on September 15, 2016, and by the end of 2021, Sarah was still off her medication and had given birth to another child. "Although I didn't enjoy the cold to start with," she says in the episode, "the effect it had was like a weight being lifted off my shoulders."

This is just one person's experience, but I cannot count the number of people who've told me that seeing Sarah's story inspired them to take up cold water swimming at least as one part of their mental health regime.

THE BIRTH OF CHILL

A full three years after the program first aired on the BBC, a surf-lifesaving coach and coast guard named Mike Morris reached out to me. Mike recognized how much good might come from running group sea-swimming courses for people with anxiety and depression.

Over tapas in Bristol, sitting waterside under the early autumn sun, we put together the rough outline for what became our "Chill Therapy" program, an eight-session swimming protocol for people with anxiety and depression. A key part of our original vision was a research component. Our intention was to collect hard data to supplement the anecdotal evidence about the benefits of cold water swimming in order to present it to the medical community. We decided to run the Chill Therapy sessions in Devon, near Mike's home, because its beaches are sheltered. This makes them safe for every kind of swimmer in nearly every kind of weather.

With his enthusiasm and energy and the support of the local medical community, Mike managed to secure a small amount of funding—just enough to run a course for fifteen people. By early 2020, we were all ready to go when the COVID-19 pandemic struck. This required us to remodel each session and how to conduct our research in accordance with lockdown restrictions and social distancing protocols.

Finally, in July 2020, we ran the first session.

I ran the team doing research, and Mike worked with the participants. He was nervous, convinced no one would turn up—or if people did, none would go in the water. To his huge relief, all fifteen people did show up and they did splash around, and all shared, in Mike's words, the "joy, excitement, and elation" of coming out to the ocean.

Even better, the success of this small pilot study on the heels of Dr. van Tulleken's BBC program led to a second round of funding and a second round of Chill Therapy courses. Following the same format, these ran from September to December 2020. In total, sixty-one people participated, and fifty-seven completed the course, which consisted of eight swims over eight weeks.

What did we find out from these two programs? As it did for Sarah, cold water swimming significantly reduced the levels of depression and anxiety among participants, and it improved their ability to function socially, both at work and at home. Most impressively, and also like Sarah, improvements in mental health remained significant even three months after each course finished.

The Chill Therapy program has been going strong and running regularly ever since. As of September 2021, over two hundred people were participating in Chill Therapy courses every week. There are now seven active Chill hubs around the country and we should be approaching twenty by the end of 2022. When Mike talks to participants, at least a third say that cold water swimming has changed their lives. One woman, Kirsty, recently sent us a wonderful—but not untypical—message along with before- and after-Chill selfies: "I was broken, properly broken. And I wanted to actually physically show you what a difference you made to me and my life. It's like magic, really. Thank you, CHILL."

THE COLD WATER SWIM CURE

In 2018–19, our research team—which is run separately from Chill Therapy and as a collaboration with Mike Tipton, Heather, and others at the University of Portsmouth—surveyed outdoor swimmers to better understand their perceptions of their health and to quantify the extent to which outdoor swimming impacted their self-reported, existing mental and physical symptoms. Conducted online through the Outdoor Swimming Society, the survey received more than seven hundred responses, and it coded symptoms into five large categories: mental health; musculoskeletal and injury; neurological; cardiovascular and blood disease; and other conditions. The results suggest the probability of outdoor swimming having "some impact" on health across all medical categories to be more than three and a half times higher than having "no impact." This number jumped to more than forty-four times higher for mental health, five times higher for musculoskeletal and injury, and more than four times higher for other conditions. Overall, we found that outdoor swimming was perceived to have positive impacts on health and symptom reductions in all categories except neurological.

No matter how cold it is,
nor how grim the weather,
simply anticipating that amazing
feeling never fails to get me
into the water in the dark
depths of winter.

In August 2004, on the morning of my first cold water dip, I didn't know that I needed the cold. I only knew I needed to swim. After a rather prolonged entrance (an approach I'm still wont to take), I gasped, I hyperventilated, I felt the shock of the cold. I definitely had a sense of heightened nervous arousal, but once I got my breath back, I gave myself up to the choppy waters. I swam out along one side of Brighton's Palace Pier, round the top, through one of the arches, and back to shore. As I settled into the experience, I started to enjoy the sensation of the cold water, the energy of the small waves, and the grand openness of a seemingly endless pool unconstrained by walls of glass and concrete. Fortunately, the effects on the kidneys and bladder didn't become fully apparent until an hour or so after I was back on land, when I felt an unexpected urge to pee.

That day, I met David for the first time. An eccentric, endearing, and intelligent man, David is the Brighton Swimming Club's "old man of the sea"; his great-grandfather was one of the club's founding members. His knowledge of the currents and conditions of Brighton's waters is encyclopedic. David kindly assured me that I would not only grow accustomed to the cold, I would become addicted to it.

He wasn't quite right. Not then, not today. I still find stepping into the water in the dead of winter uncomfortable. But I am addicted to the feeling that stays with me all day after I finish my swim. No matter how cold it is, nor how grim the weather, simply anticipating that amazing feeling never fails to get me into the water in the dark depths of winter. No matter how bad I feel when I get in, I always feel better when I get out. Those first two weeks in August became my first winter, and that first winter became seventeen years and counting.

And so it is with Sarah and Solveig and Grant and a host of other cold water swimmers you are about to meet in these pages who find this practice to be an effective therapeutic.

Since the first Chill Therapy session, I have maintained that the Cold Water Swim Cure is a self-sustaining "therapy." I am convinced that, like me, participants will get hooked on the cold and continue to engage in the activity of their own accord. It has therefore been particularly gratifying that more than two-thirds of Chill Therapy participants continue to swim on their own or with different groups three months after their initial session. The great thing about this is that not only are these people continuing to get the mental health benefits of cold water swimming, they are also enjoying the physical benefits of regular exercise. Two participants have credited the course as part of their success in losing significant amounts of weight (over 28 lbs/14 kg) and going from diabetic/borderline diabetic to normal blood sugar levels.

Over time, through official surveys and personal stories, we have been able to verify that cold water swimming offers numerous mental and physical health benefits to everyone across medical categories, regardless of gender, age, or previous health history. Our research, which I detail throughout this book, highlights not only the need to remain physically active, but also the potential of cold water swimming to support transformative improvements in health and well-being.

By sticking with the practice, to paraphrase Murdoch, cold water swimmers get through the initial shock of cold to enjoy, over time, the lifting motion of the waves, which bring to mind welcome feelings of happiness, empowerment, and liberation, and drop them, safely and surely, in a reinvigorated state of newfound health and personal well-being, right there, just on the horizon.

COLD WATER SWIMMING PRESCRIPTION

Reflect on Your Health and Expectations

Before their first swim, every Chill participant completes a questionnaire about their mental and physical health to help us understand the impact of the course.

I think this kind of exercise is helpful for anyone venturing into the cold water for the first time. Take a few moments to reflect on any health issues you may have and how they make you feel physically and emotionally. What are your expectations for your own Cold Water Swim Cure? How do you think you will feel—and how do you want to feel—after your first swim? After your second? After your tenth?

CHAPTER 2

REVITALIZING AND REJUVENATING

The Felt Experience of Cold Water Swimming

IT WAS OCTOBER 2020.

The clocks had just gone back. It was dark, wet, cold, and windy. Which, of course, made it even colder. I walked down the beach thinking I was uncomfortable, that this was unpleasant, and just for good measure, the rain being driven onto my skin was mildly painful.

Fortunately, habit and momentum got me into the water. Once I was in, I felt a familiar experience, a slightly painful one as the water rose to my waist. As I gave the rest of my body up to the intense cold, I recall expelling the same troubling thoughts and heavy emotions that had accompanied me to the beach. After a few moments, I felt my "self" return to my consciousness, and I enjoyed the varied sensations of pooling around in the water.

As I walked up the beach afterward, I felt absolutely exhilarated. *This is so amazing,* I thought, *feeling the water on my skin and the power and energy of the wind and rain on my body.* Then I suddenly recalled my negative, pre-swim thoughts and realized what a powerful reorientation had just occurred.

When we immerse ourselves in cold water, we can think of nothing else. In fact, we can't really think at all; we just become part of the moment. Water unsticks us from our repetitive thought patterns and dissolves the block that exists between our daily cares and emotional baggage and the peaceful and euphoric energy around us. By exposing ourselves to the physical, physiological, and mental experiences of an open-water adventure, we develop a greater capacity for control and balance. This allows us to successfully navigate our choppy mental currents rather than be pulled out to sea, helplessly, as on a riptide.

WATER IS MAGICAL

"To enter wild water," writes author Robert Macfarlane, "is to cross a border. You pass the lake's edge, the sea's shore, the river's brink—and you break the surface of the water itself. In doing so, you move from one realm into another: a realm of freedom, adventure, magic, and occasionally of danger."

I agree with Robert. Water is magical. The magic that is all life began in water—possibly in the dynamic environment of rock pools at the ocean's edge, where "all sorts of ammonia and phosphoric salts, light, heat, electricity" could conspire together, as Adam Nicolson wrote in his wonderful 2021 book, *The Sea Is Not Made of Water*.

Water is also very odd and very, very old. Both characteristics help explain why water is so important to life. Yet we rarely stop and think about water, an element so ubiquitous and integral to our existence that we tend to ignore its palliative benefits altogether.

As everyone knows, water is composed of two hydrogen atoms and one oxygen atom. Fundamental to its properties is how the oxygen atom has a stronger pull on the electrons than the two hydrogen atoms. This results in water's distinctive molecular shape, a little like Mickey Mouse: a single oxygen atom as the head and two hydrogen atoms as the ears. This configuration turns each water molecule into a kind of mini-magnet. Because the nucleus of the oxygen atom pulls harder on the negatively charged electrons, this part of the molecule becomes the magnet's negative pole, while the positively charged hydrogen atoms act as the magnet's positive pole.

Other similar compounds with two hydrogen atoms, like hydrogen telluride and hydrogen sulfide, have low boiling points —24°F (-4°C) and 21°F (-6°C) respectively—which means they are gases under normal circumstances. Water *should* also be a gas at the temperatures and pressures we experience on Earth, yet it only starts to boil at 212°F (100°C). The reason it remains a liquid under everyday conditions is because—due to the powerful magnetic attraction of its Mickey Mouse atoms to each other—it has a remarkably high thermal capacity. That is, it has a strong ability to absorb and retain heat.

A cosmic quirk, water's high thermal capacity offers two immediate benefits. In planetary terms, it stabilizes the global temperature. In more temperate climates, for instance, it may feel as if there's a big difference in temperature during the winter and summer, but it's actually very little in the larger scheme of things. On a smaller scale, we can get a feeling for the thermal effects of water when we consider how coastal locations tend to be warmer than inland places during the winter because the ocean gives up some of its heat.

Second, and perhaps more importantly, water's high thermal capacity is vital to maintaining life. The human body functions best within an astonishingly narrow range of temperatures: 97.5°F to 99.5°F (36.5°C to 37.5°C), a difference of just 2°F (1°C). A slightly higher temperature is good for killing infections, but the body starts breaking down at temperatures above 104°F (40°C).

In my original field of research, perioperative hypothermia, it has been shown that a drop in the body's core temperature of just 1°F (0.5°C) can result in more infections and greater blood loss because the body's immune and clotting systems become less efficient. In the water, we start to notice a loss of efficiency (and mental function) as our core body temperature drops below 96.8°F (36°C). The characteristics of water are essential to maintaining our bodies in this narrow range. When it gets hot, we get rid of heat through sweat. Because we are two-thirds water, however, we don't give up heat to the environment very easily in cold weather because air has a much lower thermal capacity than water. This is also why it feels so much colder getting into water that is the same temperature as the air.

Another consequence of the strong bonds between water molecules is the phenomenon of surface tension, which allows insects to walk or skate on water, though we crash right through the surface. It's also the reason why feathers float. On a calm day, as I swim around the head of Brighton's pier, I am sometimes treated to the beautiful, peaceful sight of a tiny feather floating calmly on the surface of the deep blue-green glassy water.

The magnetic bond between molecules also generates water's "stickiness," which helps keep us afloat. It holds waves together, provides buoyancy, and creates resistance as we swim through the water. Without resistance, our hands wouldn't be able to catch the water and propel us along. Surface tension provides the familiar sensations of simply being in water. It's why, in fact, water feels wet.

Our experience of water is intimately related to its quirky physical properties. We often hear the water before we get to it. We take the sound of water for granted and do not stop and think how it's generated. This is also related to surface tension. When water moves, particularly when a wave breaks, it generates bubbles. As these bubbles burst, they generate a pressure wave, which stimulates the eardrum and is interpreted by the brain as sound. Bubbles are also a significant part of our swimming experience—whether it's the crackle of a rough ocean or the gentle tickle of the water as our hands and arms move through it.

Water's thermal properties generate its tactile sensation, most keenly in the dynamic setting of the outdoors. When the air temperature drops, the shock and sting of cold water makes us more aware of our immediate surroundings. Water's density further presses on us and similarly heightens our awareness of our environment.

Water's unique, powerful, and dynamic properties—sound, surface tension, taste, weight, and temperature—can be experienced in one dramatic sensation as we dive through its surface or a wave crashes over us. The experience of cold water swimming is a complex interaction of physics, physiology, and psychology. How these things come together tells the story of water and its therapeutic qualities.

A REGULAR SHOWER OF WELLNESS: REORIENTATION, TRANSFORMATION, AND CONNECTION

I think the overall effect of cold water swimming is neatly and helpfully brought together into three categories—reorientation, transformation, and connection. My fellow ocean swimmer and collaborator Hannah Denton first described these categories in her paper "The Wellbeing Benefits of Sea Swimming. Is It Time to Revisit the Sea Cure?"

The experience of cold water swimming is a complex interaction of physics, physiology, and psychology.

Hannah is a counseling psychologist focused on mental health, specifically how community impacts our mental well-being. Rather than concentrating on singular treatments for specific individuals, however, she tries to involve a person's larger community and entices her patients to step into places and spaces that empower and embolden them. "I think our place in community has a big impact on how we feel," she told me. "Being linked into places and spaces that allow us to have an experience of ourselves that we feel good about can be really beneficial. Conversely, feeling ostracized, undervalued, stigmatized, and discriminated against in local communities and the community at large causes harm."

Though our medical fields are different, we both believe that cold water swimming can be an effective therapeutic for improved health and general well-being. Combined, the three categories of reorientation, transformation, and connection can cause radical changes in mind, body, and identity.

REORIENTATION

As my October swimming experience attests, a cold water swim can be reorienting. The physical and mental challenges disrupt our sense of time and space, and even of our physical bodies, taking us away from our daily lives. This distance, no matter how temporary, offers an alternate and expanded perspective on our values and issues.

We encounter water through touch, taste, smell, sight, and hearing, but our five senses do not alone explain the multilayered experience of the water's embrace. A cold bath or shower is also cold and wet, but having a cold shower doesn't reorient us or affect us emotionally in the same way as outdoor, cold water swimming.

First, even before we get in the water, there is the outdoor environment, which is a constantly changing and stimulating place. We are made all the more aware of this when we strip down to our bathing suits or, in some cases, birthday suits. Doing this, we step out of our normal social and physical environment. We move our bodies in ways we don't usually. We are also often with other people who share our joy and will look after us. All these interactions elicit strong emotional responses and are magnified by the contrast with daily life.

In addition to being out of the ordinary, cold water swimming is challenging, and that in itself is part of what gives rise to the emotions that can enhance our sense of self-awareness.

In their paper "Sensing Water," Easkey Britton and Ronan Foley note that "emotions and feelings of anxiety and being overwhelmed were not uncommon among 'new' or even more experienced swimmers, especially when experiencing a sudden sensory stimulation, body sensation, or new movements in an unpredictable and ever-changing fluid environment of the sea."

The massive change and powerful physical stimulus of the cold water keeps us from dwelling on our thoughts or overthinking, which can break the cycle of anxiety. When we come through the challenge and emerge from the water, we therefore find that our emotional state has shifted from fearful and angsty toward excited and happy.

The exhilaration, joy, and sense of achievement we feel after successfully negotiating this challenge helps develop positive associations and an improved self-image, which leaves us better equipped to deal with future everyday challenges on dry land.

The process of cold water swimming also gives us practice in coping with automatic, instinctual fear or self-preservation responses. As we learn to respond to the cold, current, and swell through controlled breathing and relaxing mindfulness techniques, we teach ourselves how to respond to any environmental condition that triggers strong emotions. In what might seem a contradictory process, this simultaneously allows us to let go and regain control in what has been described as "a regular shower of wellness."

As the mind and body adapt to the cold water, the initial challenge and anxiety about safety make way for relief, the "intense embodiment" used to describe moments in competitive sports when athletes achieve a higher awareness of their bodies and what they can do in key moments. For her paper, Hannah devised the "swim-along" interview technique, recording people's thoughts while in the water. During her interview, Naomi, a sixty-year-old personal fitness trainer, observed that, for her, "physical movement produces not quite a trance state but certainly a different state in the brain, and it is one in which my mind is a lot freer."

Cold water swimmers report that this reorienting effect, derived from overcoming the challenge, translates into a newfound ability to manage their everyday lives with confidence. My close friend Bob, a swimmer in his sixties, reflecting on his sea-swimming accomplishments, confided in me that "there have been times when I have been in a stress situation, and I can look at myself in the mirror and ask, 'What are you worrying about? You have done this, you have done that, you know? You can get through this.'"

TRANSFORMATION

I am constantly grateful to be fit and healthy. As a result, I benefit most immediately from cold water swimming's reorienting properties. Others who bravely endure painful and debilitating illnesses tend to benefit most immediately from cold water swimming's transformative properties. David, a Brighton Swimming Club member, suffers from crippling osteoarthritis. He swears he only finds relief in the cold waters off the coast of Brighton. Rob, another of my cold water swimming friends, has suffered since childhood from Crohn's disease. By adopting a daily regimen of sea swimming, he was able to improve his Crohn's disease and quit taking steroid tablets, thus avoiding the side effects of the medicine.

Having attended our inaugural Chill Therapy course, Caroline continues to swim once or twice a week. "It just keeps getting better!" she commented. "I have more resilience to stay in the water longer. I have not only begun to enjoy the swimming, but I now actively seek out time in my week to go swimming because I find it so beneficial."

In the months following the course, Caroline lost weight, dropping from a size 22 to a size 16: "I don't know how much weight because I don't have a set of scales at home, but I am no longer huffing and puffing when I walk, climb a set of stairs, or go for a walk around my village. My blood sugar levels used to be borderline high—I was seeing a diabetic nurse because I was prediabetic—whereas now they are regularly at the low end of normal. I was also borderline hypertensive. My blood pressure is now regularly one-ten or one-twenty over sixty or sixty-six."

Rather than pointing exclusively to her cold water swimming sessions, Caroline credits her transformation to the wider range of physical and mental health benefits that followed her regimen. "Cold water swimming was a wake-up call for me around how unfit I had allowed myself to become."

Other cold water swimmers take to the ocean for rehabilitation.

Candice, a forty-eight-year-old physiotherapist, started her cold water swimming practice following a series of surgical procedures to remove three tumors in her brain, two benign meningiomas and a pituitary adenoma. One meningioma was embedded in the cranial nerve that transmitted signals from her left ear, wiping out most of the hearing on that side and affecting her balance. To remove it, she endured a grueling ten-hour craniotomy, during which doctors drilled a hole in her head—"I still have a nail indentation on my forehead!"—then replaced a piece of her skull with a small slab of titanium. "I couldn't tolerate light," she recalls. "I needed to be in a dark room, and I had severe vertigo and nausea for approximately three weeks."

Next came surgery to remove her pituitary tumor, which continued to secrete growth hormones at an unsustainable clip. "I could no longer wear my wedding ring, and my face definitely changed. I kept getting a fright each time I caught sight of myself in a mirror." To inhibit the growth hormone, Candice received expensive Sandostatin injections for eight months and then had a full transsphenoidal resection, which required breaking her nose and literally draining the tumor out of her brain.

After a delay due to complications, Candice eventually had surgery to remove the third tumor through her eye socket. In total, her condition required twenty-three surgeries and a cocktail of cortisone and anti-seizure medication she needed to break free from.

"I remember the day clearly. It was end of March. Still chilly, but I felt desperate to get into the sea. We had approximately twenty minutes in twelve degrees Celsius, and I felt totally transformed. I was puffy, swollen, and sluggish prior to the swim and felt instantly less swollen and toxic. That was it!"

Within three months, her body was back in balance, and she was able to get off her cortisone pills.

"The more I swam," she says, "the more I wanted to swim. I felt humbled and empowered by the sea. She greeted me with different waves and moods and winds and tides each day. She was caring and powerful. She was able to hold my heavy body. She carried me when I was tired. She didn't let me fall. She let me float and cruise."

SKIN DEEP

The stimulation from cold water comes through our skin, the first point of contact with our environment.

The skin is primarily made up of three layers. The upper layer is the epidermis. The primary cells of the epidermis are keratinocytes, which manufacture and contain a fibrous protein called keratin that protects cells from damage and stress. Keratinocytes also give skin its waterproof properties. It is also hydrophobic; it repels water. This is why water simply runs off our bodies and how we experience the feeling of flow as we move through water.

Conscious awareness of flow derives from the physical interactions with the environment being transmitted as electrical signals to the brain. This is where the dermis, the second layer of the skin, comes in. The dermis contains blood, lymph vessels, nerve receptors, and other structures, such as hair follicles and sweat glands. Its five different types of nerve endings generate the multimodal sensory stimulations we get while in water, most notably touch, pressure, pain, and temperature, all of which are sent through the nervous system to the brain.

When exposed to cold, our cutaneous blood vessels shut down to keep the heat in and the cold out of our body's core. Blood vessels shut down so quickly that it traps blood in our skin, which prevents tissues from using oxygen. The rapidity of this effect at very low temperatures is beautifully illustrated by the "lobster phenomenon." This is my term for what happens to our skin when we get out of the water in the depths of winter. Under normal conditions, skin color is influenced by a blend of blue deoxygenated and red oxygenated blood. When we emerge from the cold, however, the red oxygenated blood, trapped in the skin, is unable to give up its oxygen to the body's cells, and so the skin is bright red.

The third and deepest layer of skin is subcutaneous tissue, which is made of fat and connective tissue. The fat content of this layer has the most important effect in the cold. A remarkably effective insulator, subcutaneous fat allows us to stay in cold water for long stretches. More generously proportioned people can stay in cold water for longer, and women can generally last longer in cold water than men, thanks to their more evenly distributed fat, which is a far more effective insulator than the classic beer belly many men develop as they age.

Candice's cold water excursions rehabilitated and rejuvenated her, and they sustained her when her tumor remnant grew back and she had to endure another series of procedures and prescriptions. "I was on cortisone once again. I was swollen and bloated once again. But I was comforted knowing that I could get in the sea and that it would help decompress my swelling. I love the initial sting followed by a slow and gentle spread of fire ice. It's a tingle and a warmth as blood gets redirected from limbs to organs. Someone described it as champagne in your veins—I like that."

CONNECTION

The physical sensation of cold is an important part of the experience of swimming outdoors. Yet the unique (and weird) physico-chemical properties of cold water cannot fully explain the experience. Otherwise, we could just fill the bath—or as some desperate enthusiasts did during the COVID-19 pandemic lockdown, a wheelie bin—with ice water.

Where's the fun in that?

I use the word *fun* deliberately.

The experience of swimming in cold water is a complex interaction between body, mind, and our physical and social environments. The reorienting and transformative benefits of swimming in cold water derive from this interaction, and this complex interaction connects us on a deeply profound level to nature and the environment, to others and ourselves.

Because swimming outdoors is a popular recreational activity both in the United Kingdom and the United States, an increasing amount of research has emerged on the potential health benefits of outdoor, water-based activities, especially in urban environments. So-called blue spaces like oceans, lakes, and rivers—as distinguished from green spaces like forests—have been shown to improve physical and mental well-being, and this is leading groups like BlueHealth, a pan-European research initiative, to examine how to promote this through the development of blue infrastructure. In one recent study, published in *Scientific Reports*, researchers found that living near, recreating in, and psychologically connecting to the natural world are all associated with better mental health. The survey collected data from eighteen countries and looked at how being in and connecting to nature impacted well-being, mental distress, and the use of depression/anxiety medication. "A measure of the degree to which people feel connected to nature," the authors wrote, "was found to be positively associated with positive well-being and negatively associated with mental distress and was, along with green space visits, associated with a lower likelihood of using medication for depression."

In 2019, *Psychology Today* published a roundup of blue-space studies from around the world. This included a 2018 Hong Kong study showing that people who regularly visited blue spaces reported greater well-being and had a lower risk of depression compared to those who didn't make such visits. Likewise, another study from Ireland found that better views of the sea were associated with lower depression scores in older adults.

A different review of thirty-five studies, led by researchers at the Barcelona Institute for Global Health, found that interacting with blue spaces improves mental health, reduces stress, and leads to greater physical activity—and that, in itself, can help further enhance well-being and reduce the risk for depression.

All this research attests to how outdoor swimming can improve health and promote healthy aging, and it's starting to quantify the transformative experiences of reorientation, transformation, and connection. This, of course, tracks with my more anecdotal research and work with the Chill Therapy program, and it is regularly celebrated by advocates and practitioners of cold water swimming. "It feels like it's easier to breathe," says Adam. "When you look at the ocean, you still have all the problems in the world, but it's just refreshing. It's easier to breathe."

As one of my fellow members of Brighton Swimming Club has said, "It's a reminder that you're alive. That's a real treat because, I don't know, sometimes you just take things for granted for a long time. Then you go in that water and it's like, *Wow, I'm here. I'm alive.*"

COLD WATER SWIMMING PRESCRIPTION

Visit the Water and Notice Your Mood

While there's more to practicing cold water swimming than simply—literally—taking the plunge, there isn't that much more to it. Still, I recommend working up to your first swim and preparing both physically and mentally.

One helpful step is to get in the habit of visiting the beach, or a local open-water spot, where you intend to swim on a regular basis.

While there, take note of how the air feels and how you respond to the water, mentally and emotionally. Take your shoes off, roll up your pants, and put your feet in. Take note, too, of how your mood changes after spending time near water. Notice if you feel better, more centered, and more rejuvenated.

Time these visits so that you are ready to start swimming in the summer, when water temperatures are more temperate. Then continue swimming through the fall, as air and water temperatures decrease and bring self-awareness to how the temperature of the water affects you.

Pick a regular day and time that works best for your schedule. In my opinion, nothing beats an early-morning swim. But since body temperatures are at their lowest when we first wake up, you may prefer the afternoon or early evening, when there's more light and our bodies, the air, and the water are warmer.

CHAPTER 3

FINDING YOUR COMMUNITY

Cold Water Swimming around the World

EVERY COMMUNITY STARTS WITH A SINGLE PERSON.

To her surprise, Sian Richardson has become the de facto leader of a casual but dedicated bunch of cold water swimmers called, rather cheekily, the Bluetits. Their mission, according to Sian, is to create a confident, capable community through cold water and swimming adventures.

"We are an informal group of mixed gender people who just like to swim together," she says. "Some carry on throughout the winter months, some don't. Some enter swimming events, some swim across the Channel, some meet every morning, same time, same place, and swim chat their way through the water. Others swim ice miles, some meet for coffee and cake, and maybe a swim or even a paddle. Our link to each other initially is the joy of challenging ourselves to putter in and around open water together throughout the year in swimsuits."

Initially, Sian was more concerned about staying in shape and enjoying a physical challenge than starting an international community of intrepid surf-breakers. In fact, the only reason she got anywhere close to the cold waters near her small Welsh town was to complete an ice mile, an official swim sanctioned by the International Ice Swimming Association in waters at a temperature of 40°F, or 4.5°C, or lower, wearing only a standard swimming kit, goggles, and one swim hat.

Back in 2003, when her five kids were aged between seven and fifteen, Sian was exhausted, and her doctor put her on antidepressants. Like many people, the medication left her feeling "numb." She asked her doctor when she would be able to come off them and was horrified by her answer: "When you feel better." At that point, as an alternative, she took up running, hoping it would help make a difference.

She didn't just do a little light jogging. Instead, she set her sights on completing an ultramarathon, or any distance longer than a traditional, twenty-six-mile marathon. "I am not much of an athlete, but I go for the extremes. I just do it very slowly."

In 2004, she ran the Cardiff half-marathon, and seven years later, she ran fifty-two miles through the Brecon Beacons, a mountain range in Wales, to Cardiff.

Then she started training for an Ironman with her daughter. After completing a half-Ironman, she signed up for a full Ironman in 2014. She wasn't surprised or even put out by the fact that she was unable to finish. "I had been feeling like rubbish for the last few months of my training and just wasn't moving forward."

In retrospect, it turned out that she needed to have both her hips replaced.

However, this wasn't immediately apparent at the time, so she took up ice swimming, since swimming put less stress on her body—though it wasn't any less extreme. "I really didn't like the sound of it. I just couldn't understand it. Until I heard about the ice mile."

Sian's first swims confirmed her reservations. She was horrified to ditch all her beloved gear, particularly her wetsuit, which had become like a second skin during her Ironman training.

Describing the experience as "horrendous" and "disgusting," she says, "I thought the water was bloody cold, and I didn't like the way it stung my skin or the way it affected my breathing. I couldn't see any point in it at all, but I had already decided I was going to do an ice mile. So the fact I didn't like the cold water initially presented me with one hell of a challenge to get from dislike to ice-mile attempt. I honestly didn't understand what could be so difficult in swimming a mile in four-degree water—until I got into thirteen-degree water without a wetsuit. That's when the penny dropped."

At the same time, she was fascinated by the effects of the cold water on her body, such as when her fingers "clawed," which is when the cold makes it hard to straighten or bring your fingers together. She noticed whether her shoulders or knees were more cold on any given day.

From her Ironman experience, she knew her swim time would be about fifty minutes. To prepare, she learned how much cold she could tolerate and how to deal with hypothermia. Although cold water swimming was unpleasant, she knew she could get through it, shivering, staying quiet, and concentrating on her body. "I could hear people around me expressing concern and wondering whether they should enlist medical help. At this point, I would put up my hand to indicate that they should leave me alone and that I didn't need help."

In contrast, her training partner, Tracey, would take off all her clothes and run around when she became hypothermic, something she did on more than one occasion, though she didn't remember one second of her actions. When I first started researching the effects of hypothermia, I read that one of the classic signs is "paradoxical undressing." I wondered if this effect was rare or even hypothetical, but I learned hypothermic (and often dead) mountaineers are regularly found naked. Tracey's aquatic experience indicates that paradoxical undressing relates mostly to cold temperatures rather than the wicked combination of cold temperatures and high altitude, which can lower a person's oxygen levels. This underlines an important caution: Always get out of the water if, after an extended period, you start to feel warm, not freezing, as this may be a sign of hypothermia.

Sian struggled to find water cold enough on the Welsh coast for an ice mile. Once she learned that no Welsh woman had ever before completed an ice mile, however, she doubled her efforts. Eventually, she came across a local farmer who told her his property featured a pond that, as a small body of water, cooled down quickly in winter. On a cold morning in February 2018, she set up a 260-foot lane and chugged through murky waters from end to end for twelve-and-a-half laps. Fifty-two minutes later—and three years after setting her initial goal—she completed her ice mile.

"As far as acclimatization was concerned, I was probably fine a year into the training, but my brain was not there. When I did take the plunge, I was very calm and enjoyed it all, and then of course berated myself for taking so long to do it. But it was all fine."

A few months later, she sailed through her hip replacements, thanks in large part (I like to think) to my working theory about cold water stress adaptation.

Prior to her ice mile, to break up the monotony of training, Sian and Tracey traveled to different swimming spots around Pembrokeshire. Whenever they emerged from the water, curious and concerned spectators plied them with question after question, most notably: *Why?*

About one in ten people decided to join them, and by the time Sian had completed her ice mile, her two-person group had grown to two hundred regular and semi-regular participants. The Bluetits were born, and they eventually included walks and runs as part of their activities.

Bluetits members don't have to swim. People come along to just sit on the beach and hand towels and hot drinks to swimmers. Some new members initially worry about body image, but as they realize that the other members don't care about or even take notice of other people's bodies, they quickly gain confidence and let go of their inhibitions.

"It is a welcoming, kind, encouraging community," says Sian.

Today, the Bluetits proudly claim more than six thousand members spread across 120 flocks, from Wales and Ireland to Australia and New Zealand. The group's inaugural "Great Tit Weekend" of September 2019 gathered a hundred Bluetits on the Pembrokeshire coast for walking, running, coasteering, crafting, yoga, food, drink, and, of course, fabulous cold water swims. "You do a bit of exercise, go into the moment, and feel better about yourself," Sian says. "All you can concentrate on is survival, but a little bit of something that scares you is good for the brain. Then, afterward, we are just herd animals being together and doing nothing other than chomping the grass."

BETTER TOGETHER

A group grows slowly over the years, two or three people at a time. The numbers don't matter, though. Any collection of like-minded people gathering in a common activity or shared interest is more than enough. This phenomenon has been demonstrated by researcher Mark Stevens and his coworkers. In a 2021 study, they found that, during the COVID-19 pandemic, when people couldn't meet in person with their sport or exercise groups, they developed more severe depression symptoms. Their conclusion was that belonging to groups that engage in physical activity can protect against depression.

Like the Bluetits, the Kenwood Ladies' Pond Association (KLPA) gathers regularly to swim in London's famed Hampstead Heath. This group is the heir apparent to the celebrated Winter Nymphs, who dove in the frigid waters of the Hampstead Ladies' Pond in the 1930s. In a 2016 video of the KLPA celebrating their aquatic adventures, several women spoke about the experience.

"It means a morning meditation," says swimmer Mary Cane in the video, "and contact with other women, which is extremely valuable. Contact with people who enjoy the same thing and contact with the wildlife and the sheer beauty of the place."

Fellow member Mary Powell said she gets "as high as a kite" when she gets out of the water, while Sarah Saunders swore that she would feel like "half the person I am if I couldn't swim in the pond."

Another KLPA member, Hilary Townley, described swimming in the pond as "beyond joy. It's life-enhancing, life-affirming. In the world that we live in, it is a beacon of light."

The Bluetits and KLPA are hardly alone.

In 2018, more than 7.8 million Englanders swam in open water and in outdoor pools, according to the Sport England Active Lives survey.

My Brighton Swimming Club has been at the vanguard of this trend for over a century, ever since a small band of swimming enthusiasts inaugurated the club on May 4, 1860, during a meeting at the Jolly Fisherman public house on Market Street. Only 13 members made up the club in its first year, a far cry from the 250 who make the most of the sea-swimming facilities today.

Current members of my club echo the Kenwood Ladies.

"It's obviously really good for you," says Jane, "and there's an extra element to it, just much more than that, an emotional well-being that you get from swimming in the sea. There's just nothing like it."

Charlotte agrees about the physical and mental benefits to swimming in the cold waters of the Atlantic, and adds, "There's a bonding experience as well. You can arrive not knowing anybody, and you get in the water and, all of a sudden, you've got a load of friends with you."

The connection with fellow swimmers is heightened by the shared experience of the water and everyone's reliance upon one another. This leads to strong and positive relationships that offer emotional support during moments of physical and mental discomfort.

While multiple studies have shown how spending time in nature and near blue spaces can reduce stress, another key to achieving better mental health and greater life satisfaction, according to recent research, is forming and maintaining relationships. A meta-analysis of 148 studies involving over four hundred thousand participants showed positive social relationships were associated with a 50 percent increase in survival, whereas poor social relationships were associated with a 29 percent increase in cardiovascular disease and a 32 percent increase in strokes.

As Sian's experience demonstrates, cold water swimmers tend to attract attention as well as people willing to join them—either informally or by joining a swim group like the Bluetits or the international Outdoor Swimming Society (OSS), which adventurer and author Kate Rew established in 2006.

Described variously as "the most magical club in the world" and "the friendliest place on the internet," the OSS gives people who love outdoor water a home and identity, from England and France to America and Australia and even to Iran and Mongolia. Members include swimmers of every age and ability, and they swim everywhere and anywhere—in rivers, lakes, ravines, public pools, oceans, reservoirs, lochs, and tarns.

OSS patron—and bestselling author of *Underland*—Robert Macfarlane agrees. "We embrace outdoor swimming's ability to slip us out of recognizable reality, into something better," he writes on the society's website. "We embrace swimming's ability to enlarge and celebrate the beauty of every day, and enhance the landscape and people we meet within it."

Just like the Bluetits, the OSS enables people to "find the others," the like-minded adventurous men and women who enjoy swimming and gathering as a community.

What started as a three-hundred-member group now proudly claims over a hundred thousand members across its various social media channels and half a million visitors to its website and partner website, wildswim.com.

While the OSS has contributed to a revival of wild swimming, both as an activity and a culture, it is still at heart about bringing people together.

"Let's be clear," Macfarlane writes, "wild swimming is about beauty and strangeness and transformation—but it's also about companionship, fun, and a hot cup of tea or nip of whisky afterwards."

LIKE A FAMILY

Whether swimming with a group or taking the plunge alone, the impact is immediate, as clear and complete as the water is cold. This is something Dan O'Connor learned when he started jumping into Lake Michigan during the early months of the COVID-19 pandemic.

"During the pandemic, it was a sort of light," he told the *New York Times*. "Everything was so dark with the pandemic and the protests and politics. Then people were like, how long are you going to do it? What are you doing it for?"

He continued his ritual for an entire year, even when the air temperature in Chicago was well below freezing. On those days when Lake Michigan was frozen, he had to break the ice with a shovel to get through to the water. After posting his daytime dips on social media, he became something of a Windy City celebrity, donning a robe with his nickname "The Great Lake Jumper" across the back.

In Brooklyn, New York, Dennis Thomas organizes wintry swims in the frigid waters off the Atlantic Ocean as president of the 116-year-old Coney Island Polar Bear Club, the oldest winter bathing club in the United States. He first started cold water swimming about thirty-five years ago, when he watched, in his words, "a bunch of old guys on the beach in bathing suits." Though other people on the Coney Island boardwalk continued on with their days, unimpressed, Dennis knew he wanted to join them. "Once I did," he told me, "I thought, 'Well, I want to do it again.'"

After being a longtime member of the club, Dennis became president in 2009. Over the years, he says, membership has continued to increase. So much so, in fact, that he implemented a lottery system to ensure the club maintains its cohesion as a group. "We had an open membership system for a long time, but it just got too crowded, and the members started to feel like strangers. We had to slow it down."

Today, the Polar Bear Club, which is most known for its New Year's Day Dip, boasts a membership of 125 people. Every Sunday, between November and April, it hosts anywhere from eighty to a hundred swimmers on a stretch of toe-tingling sand in front of the New York Aquarium, which has generously offered the group use of its facilities to change in and out of their suits and warm up after their plunge in the water, which can get as cold as 35°F (1.7°C).

Whether swimming with a
group or taking the plunge
alone, the impact is immediate,
as clear and complete as
the water is cold.

Together, club members walk to the beach and gather in a large circle. After some calisthenics—"we do a rigorous set of six or eight jumping jacks," says Dennis—they all shout an improvised chant in a military-style cadence, something like, "I don't care if the water's cold. Swimming together never gets old." Dennis's favorite is "Shrinkage comes, and shrinkage goes. Monday morning no one knows."

Once everybody's in the water, they form another circle, this time holding hands in the breaking surf, screaming and hollering together, before they all commence swimming or bathing or simply splashing water on their limbs. "It's our little ritual," Dennis says, "which has its own charm. It's very much a bonding experience, and it adds to the coherence and identity of the group."

After each swim, Dennis likes to take it all in. He usually stands on the beach for a few minutes, in whatever sun the winter sky allows to shine. "It just clears my head," he says. "We all have a lot of pressure in our lives. How to pay rent. Our job. Our relationships. But when you're in the water, you can't think about anything else. It's that cold and that intense."

He credits the club's staying power and its sustained popularity to the basic human desire to be part of something, to be surrounded by like-minded folks who enjoy the same things—even if that shared interest is splashing in near-freezing water in nothing but a bathing suit and, maybe, a pair of surf boots.

"It's not about how much you can suffer, or how much you can withstand," Dennis says. "It's about how much fun you can have.

It's camaraderie, not competition. It's about the people and kinship and, yes, the warmth. We have workers, teachers, stockbrokers, hipsters, judges, single men and women, families. So many different kinds of people show up every week. This is the only thing all of these different kinds of people have in common—each other, the weather, the beach, and the ocean. We're like a family."

COLD WATER SWIMMING PRESCRIPTION

Find Your Local Community

Cold water swimming can be done alone. It doesn't require participation in a group, but I wouldn't recommend this approach. I find the experience much more enjoyable—and much, much safer—when I do it with like-minded bathers. As you prepare for your own cold water swimming experience, I suggest reaching out to local groups who do this. In addition to introducing you to the wider community of cold water swimmers, groups often know the best swimming spots and can share specific tips and best practices.

To get started, in the Resources, see "Websites and Organizations" (page 224). One thing to consider is taking an outdoor swimming course specifically designed for swimming outdoors over short and medium distances. For instance, in Brighton, the organization Pool2Pier offers courses and technical coaching—both in the pool and in open water—and these can ease immediate concerns and ready you for taking the plunge. Similar courses are available worldwide.

CHAPTER 4

RESILIENCE AND RENEWAL

Cold Water Swimming as Lifestyle Medicine

WHAT DOES JAMES BOND HAVE IN COMMON WITH SINGLE MOTHERS?

The answer is not that they both have a "license to kill."

Rather, like Bond, single mothers live a demanding existence that requires vigilance, endurance, and the ability to solve problems on the fly while everyone else is falling apart. Like Bond, single mothers are resilient and, from time to time, require a spot of recovery and rejuvenation before they take on their next mission.

Kirsti is a single mother in her forties. On top of raising a fifteen-year-old daughter and twelve-year-old twin boys, she runs the human resources department for one of Norway's largest energy companies. That's a lot for anyone, and on the whole, she manages it very well. Every year, however, between November and February, she finds her day-to-day responsibilities overwhelming due to her *vinterdepresjon*, literally "winter depression," more familiarly known to the English-speaking world as seasonal affective disorder (SAD).

Even though 5 percent of adults in the United States experience it for more than 40 percent of the year, SAD is not considered serious enough to warrant the same kind of intervention as conditions such as bipolar disorder. It does, however, warrant an entry in the all-important *Diagnostic and Statistical Manual of Mental Disorders*, which is entitled "Major Depressive Disorder with Seasonal Pattern." Symptoms associated with the condition include feeling sad, low mood, loss of interest or pleasure in things, changes in appetite and sleep, energy loss, increased fatigue, cloudy thinking, and difficulties making decisions. At the extreme, it can even lead to feelings of worthlessness and guilt and thoughts of death or suicide.

For Kirsti, this winter depression takes the form of exhaustion, periods of low mood, and low energy. She sleeps poorly, and to cope, she tends to gorge on a menu of unhealthy foods. She also suffers from inflamed joints, which radiate pain throughout her body. For the pain, she chomps through anti-inflammatories. Though they help minimize her discomfort, they don't help her low mood or her struggle to get out of bed every morning through Norway's long, dark winter months. This combination of factors has lead Kirsti to take up *isbading*—"ice bathing"—an increasingly popular swimming practice between the months of October and May. "The first time I went in," she says, "the water was extremely cold, and I nearly screamed."

She stayed in for only a few seconds, but after the swim, she still "felt euphoric and high. I now feel much calmer when I get in, and I am no longer afraid." More than this, she has achieved something that I still only aspire to master: "In fact, I've actually begun to enjoy experiencing the shock of getting in."

Kirsti says that cold water swimming has decreased her seasonal affective disorder significantly. "I don't fall down so low," she says. "This year, I've only had three to five days with such low energy levels that I've spent the whole day lying on the sofa. Before it would have been fifteen to twenty."

Kirsti doesn't suffer from a full-blown clinical disorder, but she still needs something: a complete physical and mental reset. If there's one word that I (and others) have used more than any other to describe the effects of cold water swimming, it is *revitalizing*. Kirsti's experience illustrates the ability of cold water swimming to transform the body and the mind.

Other than James Bond—and, of course, working mothers like Kirsti—very few of us are tasked with the kind of relentless action and world-in-the-balance emergencies that define their day-to-day job descriptions. Still, even Bond can't prevent himself from falling victim to the vicissitudes of modern life. At the beginning of Ian Fleming's novel *From Russia, with Love*, Bond hasn't been on assignment for some time, and he is eloquently described as experiencing the same kind of ennui that afflicts us in the twenty-first century when we have too much screen time and seclusion, both voluntary and involuntary alike. Fleming wrote: "The blubbery arms of the soft life had Bond round the neck, and they were slowly strangling him. He was a man of war and when, for a long period, there was no war, his spirit went into a decline."

Lives spent in front of screens result in sedentary lifestyles, less human-to-human interaction, and longer hours indoors, where we face fewer physical challenges. Fast food may be convenient and cheap, but it can be terrible for the body. Eating junk food provides a brief sugar boost that feels good for a moment, a temporary boost of "happy" neurotransmitters. But these are ultimately unfulfilling and leave us craving more. While a little down time and a bit of self-indulgence are, without question, good things, too much of either results in physical and mental decline and can lead to acute and chronic lifestyle illnesses.

Unlike Bond, we don't need war to feel better, but humans are designed for physical and mental challenges.

To drag himself out of his funk, Bond performs a set of rigorous exercises. This approach is supported by science. Physical activity helps maintain both cardiovascular and mental health and reduces stress and inflammation, although we don't know whether the latter is the reason for its benefits or just an association. A study published in the *British Journal of Sports Medicine* made this abundantly clear: "Existing randomized trial evidence on exercise interventions suggests that exercise and many drug interventions are often potentially similar in terms of their mortality benefits in the secondary prevention of coronary heart disease, rehabilitation after stroke, treatment of heart failure, and prevention of diabetes."

For far too long, doctors and medical professionals have overlooked the importance of healthy eating and active living for treating chronic lifestyle issues. Thankfully, the consensus is now moving away from pharmacological interventions. Rather than considering how medicines affect lifestyle and mood, doctors and health professionals increasingly evaluate how lifestyle changes and natural interventions can be used as their own kind of effective medicines and therapies under the umbrella of "Lifestyle Medicine."

Cold water swimming is the ideal example of this approach. But before describing how it can be so effective, it's worth looking more closely at the growing pandemic of lifestyle illnesses around the world, which are afflicting nearly everyone.

THE RISE OF LIFESTYLE ILLNESSES AROUND THE WORLD

For instance, consider cardiovascular disease. This is on the rise because of modern lifestyles, which often include lots of highly processed food, low levels of physical activity, and smoking, and these multiple assaults on the body send us into a vicious cycle of ill health.

Unlike Bond, we don't need war to feel better, but humans are designed for physical and mental challenges.

Cardiovascular disease occurs when the walls of our arteries are damaged, which restricts the supply of oxygen to our limbs and vital organs. Any organ and any limb can be affected by it.

The classic manifestation is a heart attack, which occurs due to damage to the vessels supplying the heart. In 2018, heart disease was the leading cause of death in both the United Kingdom and the United States. It affected more than one in ten adults, and related conditions accounted for 27 percent of all deaths. That same year, around the world, about 18 million deaths were attributed to cardiovascular disease, an increase of 21.1 percent from 2007.

Stroke and some kinds of dementia are often the consequence of damage to the blood supply to the brain. Within a generation, between 1990 and 2016, the mean global lifetime risk of stroke increased from 22.8 percent to 24.9 percent.

When the blood supply to our extremities becomes critically low, due to the damage in the blood vessels, the body is no longer able to keep out the billions of bacteria that usually live in harmony on our skin, and significant infections can result. Low blood flow can also produce pain so severe that it cannot be treated with painkillers. In both scenarios, the only treatment option may be amputation of the affected limb.

Damage to the blood vessels is magnified by another common consequence of the typical Western lifestyle—hypertension, or high blood pressure. Hypertension increases the risk of heart failure, coronary artery disease, stroke, chronic kidney disease, peripheral arterial disease, and vascular dementia. After poor diet, hypertension is the second biggest known global risk factor for disease. In the United States, the lifetime risk of hypertension from age twenty to eighty-five is around 85 percent for adult males and black females, and 70 percent for white females. In the United Kingdom, more than one in four adults are affected by high blood pressure, and hypertension is the third biggest risk factor for disease after smoking and poor diet.

Obesity is a condition that raises the risk of hypertension. In 2016, 37 percent of all US adults, and 21 percent of young adults and children, were obese. In the United Kingdom, 64 percent of adults were overweight; of these, an estimated 28 percent were categorized as obese. Obesity also contributes to osteoarthritis, which is caused by the wear-and-tear of the joints—damage that is exacerbated in proportion to the amount of weight transmitted through them. An estimated 54.4 million US adults suffer from osteoarthritis. Notably, its prevalence is significantly higher among adults reporting no leisure-time physical activity (23.6 percent) than among those who report meeting physical activity recommendations (18 percent). In the United Kingdom, approximately one in five adults over the age of forty-five have osteoarthritis of the knee, and one in nine have osteoarthritis of the hip.

In combination, obesity, arthritis, and low physical activity create a spiral of ill health. This is exacerbated by another of obesity's many consequences, type 2 diabetes. Between 2013 and 2016, an estimated 26 million US adults were diagnosed with type 2 diabetes; around 9.4 million adults had undiagnosed diabetes; and 91.8 million Americans suffered from prediabetes. In the United Kingdom, since 1996, the number of people diagnosed with diabetes has risen from 1.4 million to 3.5 million, and another half-million people live with undiagnosed diabetes. This estimate is expected to rise to 5 million by 2025.

Diabetes is, for the most part, a lifestyle disease, one that exacerbates both hypertension and cardiovascular disease. It is also associated with its own problems, most notably reduced resistance to infections, which has particularly serious consequences for feet and legs.

All these physical issues are inextricably linked and tend to exacerbate one another. They also affect mental health. High blood pressure, obesity, and type 2 diabetes are all physical conditions that have been linked with low mood, poor motivation, loneliness, and a general sense of emptiness and lack of personal satisfaction. These mental health issues are also partly responsible for the rise in drug and alcohol abuse and the shockingly high rates of suicide. In the United States, the combination of overdose and suicide is the leading cause of death for people between the ages of ten and forty-four.

The equation is simple. If the body isn't working, it's hard to maintain a healthy mindset to rehabilitate it. And if we're mentally exhausted or depressed, it's hard to maintain our physical well-being.

THE COMMON CAUSE: INFLAMMATION

This equation is why these illnesses are often locked together in a vicious cycle: Poor nutrition and overeating lead to obesity, which over time leads to diabetes and arthritis. These, in turn, limit physical activity and make it next to impossible to lose weight, which results in low mood and little to no physical activity. This, of course, can perpetuate comfort eating and bingeing, which exacerbate diabetes and increase obesity.

We do not know all the ways lifestyle illnesses and mental health link together, but there is a common thread: inflammation.

Inflammation results from the release of a number of different chemicals by the cells of the immune system. This physiological level of inflammation is healthy and a vital part of the body's self-defense mechanism. Inflammation is a normal part of the body's healing response to tissue damage, but it can also lead to swelling and irritation and, paradoxically, when left untreated, can increase the risk of infection. If significant quantities of these chemicals are present over a long period of time—usually as a result of stress or autoimmune diseases—it can have even more negative effects. This is called "pathological" inflammation.

What happens when the body is exposed to high levels of these substances?

For a start, pathological inflammation thickens the walls of blood vessels, causing hypertension and requiring the heart to pump harder to supply blood to the vital organs, limbs, and joints. As a consequence, it's more difficult to get vital supplies to repair damaged tissues, which leads to long-term joint, organ, and tissue damage.

When the body's inflammatory system is activated and imbalanced, the result is higher levels of sugar in the blood and a disordered metabolism of dietary fat. This predisposes someone to type 2 diabetes, obesity, and infection, which creates a negative feedback loop that reduces physical activity and increases damage.

The consequences of chronic inflammation correlate with the disturbing global pattern of lifestyle-related illnesses that leave us feeling sick and tired—and sick and tired of feeling sick and tired—and in desperate need of the kind of recovery-and-rejuvenation protocol cold water swimming provides. Not only does cold water swimming produce all the benefits of exercise, it seems to magnify them, which heightens our awareness of our own body and, interestingly, creates a euphoric sense of mental well-being.

THE COLD SHOCK PROTEIN AND DEMENTIA

The underlying problem in the early stages of Alzheimer's and other forms of dementia is the loss of connections, or synapses, between nerve cells in the brain. These faulty synapses result in memory loss, confusion, mood swings, and eventually, the death of entire brain cells.

Professor Giovanna Mallucci runs the UK Dementia Research Institute at the University of Cambridge. She was intrigued by the number of animals—bears, hedgehogs, and bats, among others—that cull between 20 and 30 percent of their synapses, an enormous amount, when they hibernate for the winter. Doing so preserves the resources they require to get through hibernation. More interesting, though, was the fact that these animals reform these connections in the spring, when they awake. She and her team started looking into why and how this happens. In 2015, they discovered that this regeneration is stimulated by a specific protein—the RNA-binding motif protein 3, or RBM3—which is called the "cold shock" protein.

To explore the therapeutic benefits of this, Professor Mallucci and her team injected this protein in mice with neurodegenerative conditions. This slowed the onset of dementia, and the introduction of the protein even repaired some of the existing neurological damage. The mice also lived longer.

The next stage of their research was to see if this protein is found in humans. Rather than cool people down in a laboratory, they turned to the hardy souls who swim year-round in the Parliament Hill Lido in London, one of the outdoor pools we use for our Chill Therapy courses. Members of a local tai chi club, who practice beside the pool but never swim in the pool, provided the perfect control group. The Cambridge team found that a significant number of the swimmers had markedly elevated levels of RBM3. None in the tai chi group did.

It is notable that, during this study, the swimmers chose to stay in the water long enough to become hypothermic; their core temperatures dropped as low as 93°F, or 34°C. While I'm convinced that being exposed to the cold is good, becoming hypothermic is bad. I would therefore like to see whether increases in RBM3 levels are also seen in cold water swimmers who don't become hypothermic.

On the basis that the risks of becoming hypothermic outweigh any potential benefits, Professor Mallucci concluded that "cold water immersion is certainly not a potential dementia treatment."

I agree that cold water swimming may not be a good treatment once someone has dementia. For one, putting patients with dementia in a cold pool has its own dangers. However, prevention is better than a cure. And I contend that cold water immersion—while avoiding hypothermia—does have a potential role in the prevention of this common, distressing, and debilitating condition.

Interestingly, the "low synaptic density" seen in dementia and hibernating mammals is also seen in depression, which leads me to believe that a similar regeneration of synaptic connections through the cold shock protein could be another way in which cold water swimming improves mental health.

At this stage, this remains highly speculative. While we can see an immediate effect of cold water on mood, we need more research, following different groups in parallel over several years, to really know what the full impacts are.

Nonetheless, this provides yet another reason to experience the cold embrace of the water.

RESILIENCE AND RENEWAL

While James Bond suffers from a fictional malaise, and Kirsti suffers from a very real condition, they both benefit from a similar prescription. Cold water helps revitalize them. In the novel, after Bond finishes his exercises, he takes a shower: "Panting with the exertion, he went into the big white-tiled bathroom and stood in the glass shower cabinet under very hot and then cold hissing water for five minutes."

Taking cold showers is just one example of how Bond puts in the time and effort to develop his legendary resilience. Fortunately, this method of building resilience works in real life—as Kirsti discovered when she began a regular cold water swimming practice, which is even more effective.

Psychologists define resilience as the process of adapting well in the face of adversity, trauma, tragedy, threats, or significant sources of stress. The road to resilience inevitably involves facing distress as part of the process. While stress manifests itself in our consciousness as a psychological phenomenon and in our body as inflammation, its roots lie in our physiological responses to the environment—all those chemical messengers rushing round the body, putting our heart rate up, causing us to breathe fast and shallow, and keeping us on edge so we can deal with the next threat.

Because stress often takes the physiological form of inflammation, it makes sense that a physical riposte exists. A paper by

Jonathan Stone and his team argues that the stresses that induce resilience arise from everyday sources like sunlight, food (and lack of food), and physical exertion. At low levels, such stresses trigger a protective response. At higher levels, however, these same stresses can cause inflammation and damage tissues.

One of the most common comments I hear when I tell people I enjoy cold water swimming is "You must be mad." How, they often ask, can something as stress-inducing as cold water swimming possibly be good for you?

The answer, in a word, is hormesis, an adaptive response of cells and organisms to moderate and intermittent stress.

The concept of hormesis is often traced back to an early-sixteenth-century Swiss scientist and physician known as Paracelsus, though his rather magnificent full name was Philippus Aureolus Theophrastus Bombastus von Hohenheim. His best-known maxim roughly translates as: "All things are poison, and nothing is without poison. The dosage alone makes it so a thing is not a poison."

Basically, high doses of any substance, including water and oxygen, are potentially toxic and even lethal, but exposure to low doses can be good for us because they promote resistance and resilience.

Hormesis—a low-level good/high-level bad model—also applies to physical stresses.

The stresses that induce tissue resilience, as Stone and his team underline, arise from everyday sources, most notably ultraviolet radiation from the sun. Essential to our production of vitamin D, ultraviolet light can, at low levels, improve cardiovascular health, enhance resistance to cancer, and improve immune function, mood, and sleep. Conversely, at high levels, such stresses cause tissue destruction. In the case of ultraviolet light, these stresses include sunburn and, at the extreme, malignant melanoma.

Similarly, excessive exposure to cold leads to hypothermia, but moderate and intermittent exposure to cold allows us to withstand the stress, which produces positive health benefits and gives us the confidence and physical and mental ability to endure other stresses in the future.

In addition to Stone's work, reports of stress-induced resilience can be found in journals dedicated to the fields of neuroscience, sports medicine, cancer, healthy aging, dementia, Parkinson's disease, and even ophthalmology. The benefits of stress-induced resilience include faster wound healing and a demonstrable slowing of age-related degeneration in the brain and other nervous tissue, muscles, and bones. Stress-induced resilience has also been shown to suppress certain kinds of cancers. Basically, a whole raft of physiological effects can contribute to a longer and healthier life—all through exposure to the kinds of stresses that cold water swimming presents, namely exercise, exposure to the elements, and physical challenges.

A recent study published in *Experimental Physiology* showed that swimming exercise decreased depression-like behavior in diabetic mice by reducing inflammation. Swimming, according to the authors, is associated with both an improvement in mood and a reduction in inflammation, which indicates it might be a useful treatment of depression-related disorders in patients with type 2 diabetes. I would qualify their findings by pointing out how swimming in *cold* water is likely to enhance this effect.

At first, it might seem somewhat paradoxical to willingly expose ourselves to a challenge like swimming in a winter ocean, when the air is also cold, the weather often intemperate, and the sun barely a rumor in the gray sky. Many people might regard this as something to be avoided at all costs. However, voluntary risk-taking can bring some overlooked benefits. For instance, it builds character, which increases self-esteem and enhances psychological resilience, and these can be translated into every other area of a person's life. Undertaken with an appropriate degree of caution and a *healthy* sense of fear, cold water swimming offers a controlled, safe, yet exciting challenge. It's an ideal environment in which a person can experience—and grow accustomed to—moments of stress.

CHILL OUT: EMBRACE THE COOL TO STAY COOL

This link between high levels of inflammation and both physical illness and poor mental health is what led to my "that's funny" moment when I came up with the theory that cold water swimming could help treat depression.

Sitting in my favorite pub one evening, defrazzling from a day of work with a pint and a copy of the *Guardian*, I came across an article titled "Is Depression a Kind of Allergic Reaction?" It posed the question: "If people with depression show classic sickness behavior and sick people feel a lot like people with depression—might there be a common cause that accounts for both?"

Of course, as this chapter describes, the answer is inflammation, and it is worth considering what causes inflammation and, more importantly, how cold water swimming might be able to influence it to ward off physical ailments and mental malaise.

Because (good) inflammation is predominantly a process that defends and repairs the body, the main cause of inflammation is infection and injury. In this context, it is an appropriate response. However, this response, which is mediated by the body's autonomic nervous system, can also be produced by low levels of chronic stress. Unlike infection and injury, inflammation is not an appropriate response to chronic stress. In the past, the traditional medical orthodoxy was that the autonomic nervous system, since it functions autonomously, is not a suitable target for medical interventions. Thankfully, this view is changing, due largely to emerging research that has documented the success of practices like breathing techniques, meditation, and yes, cold water swimming to impact it.

Broadly, the human nervous system is divided into two parts: the somatic and the autonomic. We have conscious control over the somatic nervous system, which includes the body's musculoskeletal system; thus, we can control our fingers, feet, and how our body moves. The autonomic nervous system operates automatically, without conscious direction; thus, our hearts beat and lungs breathe without being told.

The autonomic nervous system is further divided into two parts, the sympathetic and parasympathetic, both of which are in opposition to each other. Ideally, this tension creates a harmonious balance, regulating a healthy response to stress and other stimuli. They act a bit like Dr. Doolittle's pushme-pullyu, constantly struggling against itself. During times of stress, the sympathetic system pulls hardest, which leads to the fight-or-flight response. This causes rises in heart rate, blood pressure, blood sugar, and inflammation, among others. During times of rest (and digestion), conversely, the parasympathetic system pulls hardest, which resets the body and reduces inflammation. Much of its activity is mediated through the vagus nerve, which arises from the brainstem. To help reset the body, the parasympathetic system diverts blood away from the muscles to the gut to aid digestion and to stimulate salivation and gastric acid secretion. It also slows the heart rate and reduces blood pressure. Importantly for general health and well-being, stimulation of the vagus nerve and the parasympathetic nervous system reduces levels of inflammation in the body, which results in better health and gives our body some much-needed recovery time, particularly in today's always-on culture.

Modern lifestyles result in a lackadaisical parasympathetic nervous system working against an irritable and sensitive sympathetic nervous system, which leaves us susceptible to stress and dangerous levels of inflammation. For optimal health, both systems need to be strengthened, toned, and effectively balanced.

This is where cold water comes in, since it engages both the body's sympathetic and parasympathetic nervous systems. Whether it's James Bond in his white-tiled shower or Kristi plunging into Norwegian fjords, both get a sympathetic boost from the cold. Then, once they have adapted to the cold, and the resultant sympathetic boost is reduced, they enter into a more autonomically balanced physiological and mental equilibrium. After repeated exposure to cold water, their bodies' response attenuates, and their nervous systems no longer overreact to subsequent stresses or any other daily challenge. This leaves Bond and Kristi—and you and me and every other cold water swimmer—less sympathetically charged in normal moments, when there's absolutely no need to be keyed up.

This is why cold water swimming leaves us feeling rejuvenated and resilient, less blah or sickly or susceptible to low moods. While it boosts our sympathetic nervous system when we're in the moment, leaving us with that euphoria, in daily life it runs at a healthier level and helps prevent lifestyle illnesses. Then, when we put our face in the water, our parasympathetic nervous system kicks in, which helps recalibrate our bodies' natural resting state and helps bring down the concentration of inflammatory chemicals to healthier levels—so we feel more like ourselves, our best selves.

Think of it this way: We all need to chill out sometimes, even James Bond and especially single mothers of three, and a great way to do so is by, literally, chilling out.

COLD WATER SWIMMING PRESCRIPTION

Take a (Mini) Plunge

Recently, I led a group of high school students in Norway in a quick cold water immersion activity. As part of our preparation, I invited them to dunk their faces in an ice bath and, as a companion practice, to stick and keep their hands in ice water. These activities elicited an enthusiastic response from the students, and it demonstrated to them how these "interventions" kick-start their parasympathetic and sympathetic nervous systems respectively.

You can do the same thing by way of preparation for taking up cold water swimming. Put your face into a bowl of ice water. You don't have to submerge your entire head. You may not be able to hold your breath on the first occasion but try it a second and third time to get acclimated. Be prepared for an initial shock, but try and keep your face in the water for a few seconds until the worst of the discomfort has passed.

You can also submerge your hands in ice water, which will give you a sense of how your extremities will respond to a cold water plunge and help your body start to adapt to this stress.

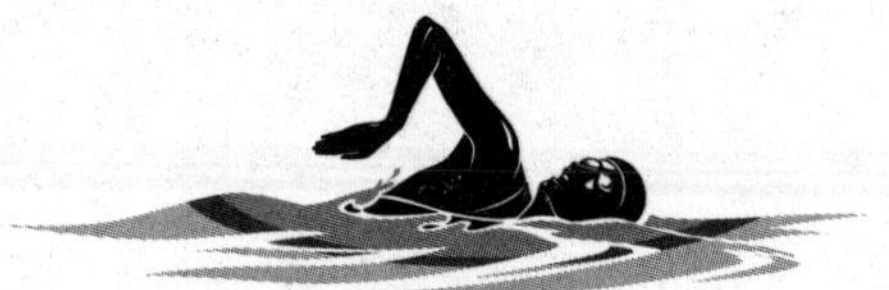

PART II

The Cold Water Swim Protocol

CHAPTER 5

GETTING STARTED

Preparing for Cold Water

THE FIRST SWIM IS THE MOST TERRIFYING. But the excitement and adrenaline always carry you through.

The second swim is the worst: You know what to expect, so you are not as distracted from the cold, but you aren't used to it either.

The third swim teaches you how to start enjoying it.

The first time I noticed this sequence was with Sarah when we were filming the BBC program with Chris van Tulleken (see "A Soothing Swim," page 224). Sarah did great on her first swim, but after her second dip, she was reluctant to carry on with the project. On her third time in the water, however, she fell in love with it. Swimming in cold water was no longer a problem.

Initially, I dismissed this as a one-off event, something unique to Sarah and her personality and circumstances. Then in the winter of 2020, my eleven-year-old son, Ib, decided to join me for cold water swimming. My son followed the same trajectory as Sarah. After enduring the first swim, he was perfectly happy coming with me on a second swim, but after that dip, he flat-out refused to do it again. Eventually, the lure of extra screen time proved strong enough for him to go for a third swim. Since then, he's always eager to check the temperature of local waters, especially when we need to cut a hole in a frozen lake with a chainsaw.

Actually, the truth is, I've found that full acclimatization to cold water swimming takes up to six dips, so if you have never done this before, I recommend committing to at least that many. Give yourself time to get used to the experience before making up your mind whether to continue.

On the face of it, cold water swimming is simple. You just swim and in exactly the same way you'd swim in any body of water. Knowing how to swim is the only genuine requirement.

That said, there are three things to do as you prepare for your first cold water adventure:

1. Set a place and time to swim
2. Find a friend
3. Get appropriate equipment

MAKING PLANS: FIND WATER, SET A SCHEDULE

Initially, I recommend making a cold water swim plan that includes six swims at a fixed time, a fixed place, and with a fixed partner or group. Coupled with a firm plan to get a hot drink afterward, this is the best way to prevent procrastination or, worse, cancellation. After completing one of our Chill Therapy courses, Grant (who is featured in chapter 7) remarked that one of the best things about it was the shared exhilaration and laughter: "Everyone was instructed to bring a thermos so they could prolong this positive sense of community."

Ideally, swim outside in a natural body of water. If you live close to a coastline, swim in the ocean, as I do. However, a lake, pond, or slow-moving river is also great. Choose public locations that are already used for swimming, since these tend to have the safest access points. If no natural water is suitable or close enough to be convenient, then locate an outdoor pool.

Arrange to swim at minimum once a week. Any less than one swim per week risks losing the adaptive changes. The good news is, I find the more frequently I swim, the easier and less discomfort I have getting in even the most frigid waters in the middle of winter.

To reduce the initial discomfort, I suggest starting in the middle of the summer. That's what, quite by chance, I did. The coastal waters surrounding the United Kingdom and Ireland remain uncomfortably cold even in summer, when maximum water temperatures reach around 68°F, or 20°C. That's cold enough to provide the full beneficial effects of cold water adaptation. But even if you're blessed to live where ocean waters are warmer in summer, simply carry on swimming through the fall and into winter. By the time the water gets really cold, you will have gotten into the habit and—as David said to me when I started out—quite likely have developed an addiction to it.

Pick a time of day that works best for you and your schedule. Much as I love the peace and quiet of a morning swim, our body temperatures are naturally at their lowest at this time of day. Regardless of the season, the water will also feel less cold if you swim in the afternoon or evening. Swimming in the afternoon adds the benefit of more light and the radiant warmth of the sun. I even notice a big difference between my usual time of around 6:45 a.m. and the odd occasions when I swim at 10 or 11 a.m.

FIND A FRIEND OR SWIM GROUP

When swimming outdoors, it's imperative you do it with other people. This is of tantamount importance to your safety. Because open water is not a controlled environment, there is always an element of risk attached. A feeling of risk actually enhances the experience, but minimize real risk by having company.

Ideally, you can convince a friend to swim with you, but even if no one wants to join you in the water, bring someone to watch from dry land. That way, if there's an emergency, they can get help. Plus, nothing enhances the postswim high more than sharing the exhilaration, joy, and laughter with others.

You can also seek out a local cold water swim group or club. Many communities have them. In addition to motivation and camaraderie, groups can provide information about, and sometimes access to, the best swimming spots, and they can share specific tips and best practices beyond the ones in this book. Swimming clubs may even have welcome facilities, including a locker room or sheltered space to change and shower.

Another advantage of clubs—at least for those who are ambitious and experienced enough to confidently swim significant distances outdoors—is that they sometimes offer outdoor swimming courses that provide technical coaching, both in the pool and in open water. A great example of this is the Pool2Pier course in Brighton. For more than a decade, their course has introduced hundreds of people to the ocean, including many who subsequently joined my Brighton (swimming) club and now swim round the pier with me on a regular basis.

To help find a local group near you, check out "Websites and Organizations" (page 224) under Resources. Some are volunteer-led, like Mental Health Swims (for more, see "Mental Health Swims: Rachel's Cold Water Swim Cure," page 188) and the Bluetits, which has become something of a phenomenon, with affiliated groups on both sides of the Atlantic. Similarly, the Outdoor Swimming Society helps connect like-minded cold water swimmers around the world. Our own Chill Therapy program is more formal, so the key is learning what's available near you and finding the right group for yourself.

A PROPER SWIM KIT: EVALUATE YOUR EQUIPMENT

Before you take the plunge, make sure you have a proper kit for cold water swimming. Of course, some people don't feel the need for any kit at all—as a picture of one of my friends in a national newspaper proved. The caption under the infamous nude photo read, "Chilly round the willy." This is not an approach I advocate. In fact, some people like to wear a second swimsuit over the first, which takes a little bit of the initial cold shock off the more sensitive areas.

Here are some other items you might consider:

- A thick, brightly colored swimming cap
- A pair of swimming shoes
- A pair of neoprene gloves
- A wetsuit

Personally, after a swimsuit, I believe the only essential piece of equipment is a brightly colored swim cap. This keeps your head warm and it helps make you visible to other swimmers and to boats. The other items are great options when starting out and can be necessary in certain circumstances.

Contrary to popular belief, we don't lose 95 percent of our body heat through our head. This figure came from a study where the rest of the body was encased in an immersion suit. Proportionately, however, we do lose a greater percentage of heat from our head because it is poorly insulated and the blood vessels in the scalp do not close down like they do over the rest of the body when we're immersed in cold. Rather than a swim cap, some swimmers prefer a woolly bobble hat or beanie, but only use these if you are going to put your face in the water rather than your entire head.

Footwear can be helpful for several reasons, and in winter, I always swim with something on my feet. First, many wild swimming spots have rocks and/or other uncomfortable ground features, so a pair of shoes helps navigate such terrain. Then, having footwear means it's not actually physically painful to put your feet in the water. Finally, when the waves or surf are a bit rough or marginal, shoes provide extra grip on the shore, which allows you to stay ahead of the incoming waves with greater confidence and more stability as you extract yourself from the water.

What kind of footwear is best? For many years I used wetsuit shoes—just light summer ones because they do a good enough job and are much easier to take on and off than thicker and warmer ones. But I find them awful to swim in. Then, during 2020, I visited a friend in Cornwall. Because we had to walk about three miles to our swim, he lent me a pair of "aqua trainers"—basically a light running shoe base with a mesh upper that is designed to get wet. These rewarded me with a much more enjoyable swim. I barely noticed I was wearing them. Even better, I could walk or jog in them after swimming, so I didn't have to waste any time in the cold getting them on and off.

I also don't like swimming gloves, but when the water temperature dips below 50°F, or 10°C, I put on a pair. I swim outdoors for fun, not for pain. That said, no matter how much I tape them up, even using swimming-specific gloves, I find they quickly fill up with water. I consider them a necessary evil in colder temperatures.

Finally, I personally dislike the fuss of getting a wetsuit on and off along with the inconvenience of carrying it around. I would much rather deal with the initial discomfort of the cold than lose the feeling of the water running across my skin. I'd rather swim for a shorter time without a wetsuit than swim longer with one.

Also keep in mind that while a wetsuit mitigates the cold, that also mitigates the physiological effects of cold water swimming. The body's reaction to cold is dependent on both the absolute temperature of the water and the rate of cooling, and this is lessened in a wetsuit. This is also why cold showers—while they have been shown to have certain benefits—are not as effective as full-on bodily immersion.

That said, some people need a wetsuit just to get into the water, and if that's the case for you, wear one. Rest assured that you will still experience the benefits of cold water swimming, though they might not be quite as dramatic.

One more thing: Don't forget to bring towels and dry clothes to change into after your swim. For more on this, see "Rule 5: Get Out, Get Dry, and Get Warm," page 109.

TOW FLOATS

Tow floats are a bit of a contentious issue. These are inflatable devices that attach to a belt via a thin rope and drag behind while you swim. There's no doubt they increase your visibility in the water, and many have the added convenience of containing pockets in which to stash keys and even clothes, but they can be a positive hazard during mass swims, when they can get caught up in each other and drag people down.

However, it is important to note that they are not designed to be lifesaving devices like life vests. The vast majority are not sufficiently buoyant to actually hold the weight of a grown person, which means they're not a reliable safety aid.

They also get in the way of your swimming stroke. I like to be as unencumbered as possible (within the realms of decency), so I very rarely use them and will actively avoid organized swims that require them.

That said, if being visible is a high priority, or tow floats provide you with the confidence to do a cold water swim, they are very effective.

CHAPTER 6

SIX RULES FOR A SAFE AND ENJOYABLE COLD WATER SWIM

DO YOU HAVE YOUR COLD WATER SWIM PLAN? Is your kit ready? Do you know where and when you'll swim and with who? Perfect. All that's left is to swim!

As I say, cold water swimming is really simple, but that doesn't make it easy. It's unlike almost any other endeavor. You don't swim the same way you might in, say, Hawaii or the Caribbean or a backyard pool in August. Here are my six rules for a safe and enjoyable cold water swim:

Rule 1: Before you get in, know how you are getting out

Rule 2: Warm up before you get in

Rule 3: Get your body in before your head

Rule 4: Focus on your breathing

Rule 5: Get out, get dry, and get warm

Rule 6: Better together—swim with a friend

RULE 1: BEFORE YOU GET IN, KNOW HOW YOU ARE GETTING OUT

Agnes Allen gives us the first rule of outdoor swimming, which also applies to pretty much every other undertaking in life: "Almost anything is easier to get into than out of."

Long before I heard Agnes's rule, it was illustrated to me at an annual Christmas Day Brighton Swimming Club dip in the early 2000s. On that morning, years before outdoor swimming became a "thing," I was shocked by the sight of hundreds of people who had turned up to watch.

It was a beautiful day, but very windy. At high tide in Brighton, the beach shelves steeply. When the wind approaches 20 mph, it creates a dangerous shore dump, or a set of large waves often referred to as "Pirate Captain's Daughters." If you mess with them, the saying goes, you're dead. Just one cubic meter of water weighs, literally and by definition, a tonne. Thus, a single, badly timed wave can crush a swimmer into the shingle. In addition, the force of the waves generates a churn at the edge, affectionally referred to as the "washing machine," which can trap swimmers and tumble them over and over, keeping them from getting onto shore.

On this occasion, my fellow club members and I stood at the edge of the ocean and judged this year's swim too dangerous.

However, two or three of the onlookers decided to risk it. Clueless as to the difficulties of getting out of such turbulent waters, they were lucky to survive, and they did so only thanks to the efforts of experienced swimmers from the club.

In 2019, I was asked to explain the benefits of outdoor swimming on the UK television program *This Morning*. Of course, this was to be filmed on location, and on this occasion the venue was the River Ouse, where the swimming itself was organized by a local group. When I expressed my concern about how we would get in and out of the river—especially as the inexperienced presenter would be joining us—the organizer told me not to worry: She was bringing along a specially adapted ladder, basically a standard wooden ladder cut down to fit in the back of a car but long enough to reach the bottom of the river. This did the trick perfectly and the filming was completed without incident.

More recently, during the winter of 2021, I had my first experience of proper "ice bathing" in a frozen Norwegian lake. To enter the water, a friend's father cut a hole in the inches-thick ice with a chainsaw. As I walked over the ice in my swimming trunks, I remained somewhat concerned about the sharp edges of the hole and questioned my ability to get enough purchase on the ice to pull myself out. My fears, though, were once again assuaged by the sight of a ladder emerging from the almost frozen (32.5°F/0.3°C) water.

All of this is to say, if in doubt about your ability to get out of water, only get in if you can keep your feet on the ground.

Even then, proceed cautiously, especially in moving water like rivers and oceans. Unseen objects often float just under the surface. In the ocean, tides and storms can move the seabed around from day to day and even shift heavy objects like concrete blocks. Although they may not interfere with your swimming, they can damage your feet and legs as you stride into the depths.

No matter where you're swimming, always make sure to check your exits before you enter the water.

RULE 2: WARM UP BEFORE YOU GET IN

It's a bit of a myth that you shouldn't get into cold water when you are warm because the contrast in temperatures will cause your body to go into shock.

I bought into this during my early days in cold water. I still remember cycling along the seafront one late autumnal morning. Neither the weather nor the water were particularly cold. Still, as I approached the pier, I realized that I was underdressed for the conditions and, in contrast to my usual experience, was getting colder rather than warmer. I recall thinking, *It doesn't matter because the sea is cold, and I will just be attuned to it.* I was wrong. Normally, I am aware that the air is cold as I walk down the beach, but on this occasion, I felt uncomfortably cold inside myself. And when I launched myself into the water, rather than perking up after a minute or so, I just declined steadily and got out shortly after. I should add that, even though my experience of this particular swim was unpleasant, by the time I'd warmed up I experienced the customary positive effects. This illustrates the principle that almost any swim is a good swim.

In any cold environment, the most important thing is to maintain your core body temperature as close to its optimal range of 97.7 to 99.5°F (36.5 to 37.5°C) as possible.

When you get in the water, while some of the blood from your skin remains trapped (causing the lobster effect I mention earlier), the rest is squeezed into your core. The colder that blood is, the colder your core becomes. What you want is for the blood going into your core to be as warm as possible. Imagine—as I sometimes need to do in an emergency situation—squeezing a bag of blood straight from the fridge into someone's body. That's going to create much more of a shock than squeezing a bag of nice, warm blood. The experience is analogous to having an ice-cold shower from the inside-out.

In fact, I've researched this as an anesthesiologist. One of the most effective ways to keep patients warm during surgery is to use special heating devices to warm intravenous fluids and blood as they are infused into the body.

The other factor is the second law of thermodynamics, which (in one form) says that heat flows naturally from an object at a higher temperature to an object at a lower temperature. The rate of flow is proportional to the gradient, so the colder your periphery, the quicker you will lose heat from your core.

BRAGGING RIGHTS: HOW COLD IS IT?

I can't think of a single outdoor swimmer who isn't obsessed by the temperature of the water. Obviously, I include myself in this category—to the extent that part of my PhD thesis related to temperature measurement.

A good part of this is bragging rights: The colder the water, the better the story. So if you want to quantify how cold the water is—whether for pride, entertainment, or science—you need another piece of equipment: a thermometer.

Ideally, get a thermometer that is calibrated to an accuracy of +/-0.2°F (+/-0.1°C). Unfortunately, these are expensive. Despite the fact that digital thermometers show the temperature to one decimal point, the most affordable waterproof ones only have a quoted accuracy of +/-1°F (+/-0.5°C), and many others have only a quoted accuracy of +/-2°F (+/-1°C). So it's important to check the specifications before you buy one.

The variability in accuracy is also why, if you want to swim an officially recognized ice mile, you have to check the water temperature with three thermometers.

The other specification to look out for is the equilibration time—in other words, how long it takes to give a reading. This is important when, say, you are holding the thermometer in the water while standing among breaking waves.

Avoid infrared, noncontact thermometers. These only measure surface temperature, which is as much an indication of air as water temperature.

The available nondigital thermometers are filled with alcohol, but alcohol is not stable enough for a reliable, accurate measurement. They are fine for ambient and approximate temperatures, but they cannot be considered suitable for the outdoor swimming obsessive.

This is why the old theory—that the warmer the body is, the greater the contrast with the cold water, and therefore the bigger the cold shock—doesn't hold.

The way you warm your body up before getting into cold water is also important.

If you warm up from the outside-in—such as by sitting in the car with the heater on before swimming—you will actually lose heat faster when you start swimming than if you hadn't warmed up at all. External heat sources warm the surrounding air, so the signals sent by your thermoreceptors to the brain makes it think you are warm and it behaves accordingly. However, blood just below the skin's surface remains cool or cold, and when this blood gets pulled into your core, it cools you down and confuses your temperature regulatory system.

Conversely, if you warm up from the inside-out through exercise, you will slow down the cooling process, giving you more control of your environment and core temperature.

I usually cycle to the beach for my swims, and on the occasional days when I drive, I notice that the water feels colder and getting in is more uncomfortable.

In Norway, I chaperoned a group of schoolchildren on a cold water swim. Leading up to the excursion, I instructed the students to wear warm clothes over their swimming gear. Then that morning, before we entered the water, we slowly jogged as a group about one and a half miles from their school to the local lake. Afterward, they were absolutely fine. None of them were even shivering despite being unacclimated. To warm back up, they just walked, rather than jogged, back to school.

Of course, Scandinavians like to use an external heat source in the form of a sauna to warm up prior to icy dips. We did this when I went ice bathing in the frozen lake. What happens in a sauna is that your body becomes completely "saturated" with warmth, and all your blood is warm. That is why it didn't feel too bad when I finally got in.

An alternative practice for warming up includes breathing techniques. One form, known as tummo breathing, has been championed by Wim "the Ice Man" Hof. Developed through the Tibetan Kagyu tradition, tummo breathing is a meditation technique that combines breath work and visualizations. For example, practitioners visualize a candle radiating heat from their abdomen and expanding its intensity to spread heat across their entire body. In the spiritual tradition, the heat rises and becomes more brilliant with every breath, ultimately reaching the crown of the head. It seems both doable and effective—and there's no doubt it enables Wim Hof to undertake the most remarkable feats.

However, tummo breathing is a very powerful technique and should be undertaken with caution. I asked an experienced yoga and breath work teacher about this, and she said it is important to be sensitive to how the body responds, since this kind of technique can increase anxiety. Breathing can certainly increase energy in the body, but it would be counterproductive if it increased anxiety in the face of a challenging environment.

Finally, if you become a regular cold water swimmer, you might experience what's called "anticipatory thermogenesis." This has been documented dramatically in cold water endurance swimmer Lewis Pugh.

Before undertaking swims in both the Arctic and Antarctic, Pugh's core temperature rose by 3.5°F, or 2°C. Scientists have credited this spike to a Pavlovian response to cold water swimming, while Pugh has chalked it up to fear and adrenaline.

Anticipatory thermogenesis is less a technique than a bodily response. It has yet to be officially documented in any other human, but I can personally attest to the body's ability to increase its core temperature. Prior to a six-mile swim in the River Thames, I swallowed a capsule that measured my core temperature. This recorded a change of around 1.8°F (1°C) in the time just before I got in. I suspect Lewis Pugh is exceptional in how many degrees his core temperature can raise, but my experience leads me to believe that anticipatory thermogenesis is a common ability among regular cold water swimmers.

RULE 3: GET YOUR BODY IN BEFORE YOUR HEAD

There are two main approaches to getting in: fast or slow.

For the most part, this is entirely a matter of personal preference. For instance, I'm a bit of a lightweight, and even after all these years, I still don't like getting into cold water. I therefore approach it slowly in the possibly vain hope that this will minimize the unpleasantness.

Depending on the water temperature, getting in can go from being a little uncomfortable to quite painful. In fact, one of the most common techniques for studying pain is to have subjects put a hand in ice water. One such study showed that swearing reduced a person's perception of pain. This study won a 2010 Ig Nobel Prize, which is awarded to achievements that first make people laugh, and then make them think. According to the study, it only worked for people who were nonhabitual swearers, so cursing is only effective for polite swimmers. A follow-up study calculated the frequency of habitual swearing above which the analgesic effect was lost.

Go slow and curse, or run in and scream. Just don't dive in headfirst. Enter feet first and submerge your body at a comfortable pace, keeping your head out of the water until you have brought your breathing under control.

It takes time for people to become comfortable with their heads under cold water, but this is also important from a safety perspective. First, because of the "inspiratory gasp" reflex and hyperventilation, if you put your head under before you have adapted, you risk inhaling water into your lungs. Second, in extremely rare cases, sudden immersion of your face can simultaneously stimulate the sympathetic nervous system and the fight-or-flight response as well as the parasympathetic rest-digest system. When these are in conflict, it can result in abnormal and singularly unhelpful electrical activity in the heart.

GOING UNDER: DUCKS AND DOLPHINS

Learning to get your head under the water brings confidence, makes dealing with waves safer, and quickly becomes a lot of fun. In fact, once you've practiced going under in a controlled fashion and have become adapted, it's fine to go in headfirst.

Teaching these techniques is a key part of the Chill Therapy course. But as Mike Morris says, it's "bloody difficult to explain and should be accompanied by a diagram!" Besides, if you aren't confident, it is probably best learned under supervision. Here is an explanation of the two basic techniques:

1. The dolphin dive: This is a technique to get through the surf and help avoid getting "bashed" by incoming waves. Only do this after you've entered the water and acclimatized your body. Then, as a wave approaches, dive under it with your hands over your head stretched forward in a dive position. Use your hands to pull yourself along the seabed so you have more purchase to get further out into the ocean. While underwater, breathe out. When you

reach the surface, take a quick breath and repeat until you are past the breaking waves.

2. The duck dive: We use this technique in the Chill Therapy program to give participants the confidence to overcome their fears and immerse themselves completely. This is best used when you're in water above your head, and it uses the weight of the body to take you underwater and down to the bottom. First, put your hands above your head in a dive position. Then, in a pinwheel motion, swing your arms forward so that your head is facing down, toward the bottom, and your legs swing up and out of the water. Keep your legs straight above you and point your toes, and let the weight of your legs propel you down until you reach the bottom. Then reverse position and swim back to the surface.

RULE 4:
FOCUS ON YOUR BREATHING

Cold water takes your breath away. It almost always causes hyperventilating in a way that feels very much like a panic attack. Note this. Stick with it. And know that it will pass very soon.

Once it passes, you can get out of the water if you want. To get the benefits of cold water swimming, you don't need to be in the water for a long time. You don't even have to swim. In fact, many people will just bathe or bob in a specific spot, which is affectionately known as "dipping," until hyperventilation passes.

I think the most important thing is to stay in the water long enough for your breathing to come under your conscious control again. This corresponds with the length of time required to get the benefits of a cold water swim. I said this to Kirsti when she started organizing her coworkers for a weekly cold water swim, and she said it's been the single most useful piece of advice she's heard when it comes to introducing new people to the joys of the cold.

Once your breathing is under control, another important thing to do is to put your face into the water to generate that anti-inflammatory, parasympathetic response. This doesn't have to be your whole head; you don't have to submerge entirely underwater. Despite an initial jolt of discomfort, hold your face in the water for a few seconds until the shock has passed. Do this three times.

Typically, I suggest that people stay in the water for at least three minutes, but personally, how long I spend in the water varies massively. In the summer, when the coastal water around the

UK is cold but not frigid, I might spend an hour or more. Once the water temperature dips to around 51 to 53°F, or 11 to 12°C, I can just about comfortably manage a quick dash of about fifteen minutes, swimming around the pier at low tide. By the time the thermometer drops below 46 to 48°F, or 8 to 9°C, I'm down to five minutes or so—maybe ten minutes, if the waves are good. When I was ice bathing in a frozen Norwegian lake, I lasted only for those three crucial minutes—possibly less. No matter how long or short I stay in, however, I still feel fantastic for the rest of the day. I've actually noticed that, despite only brief contact with the water, the buzz when the temperature is really low is still greater than longer, warmer swims.

To me, this indicates that the main gains occur during those first few minutes in the water.

Of course, the longer and more vigorously you swim, the more exercise you get, which is always a good thing. And some people stay in longer because they are simply having so much fun. Certainly, I find that I tend to stay in longer when the winds are up and I'm playing among the breaking waves with all the joy of a little kid. "We don't stop playing because we grow old," George Bernard Shaw wrote; "we grow old because we stop playing."

RULE 5:
GET OUT, GET DRY, AND GET WARM

During your initial swims, remember to start short, stay shallow, and keep warm.

Observe your body's response to the water, and get out before your insides get cold. How long this takes will vary depending on the changing conditions and the characteristics of each dip.

A good sign that it's time to get out is the appearance of "claw fingers." This refers to the feeling that it's difficult to bring your fingers together as you draw your hand through the water with your swimming stroke. This is a good sign to watch out for because it occurs early, and so it gives you plenty of warning to get out safely before developing hypothermia (see "Hypothermia," page 114).

Armed with this knowledge, you can safely and gradually build up the length of time you spend in the water. Over time, you will come to recognize your body telling you it's time to get out without even thinking about it.

Once you are out of the water, immediately get dry and get out of the wind and cold.

Air is a very good insulator. But to be effective at reducing heat loss, it needs to be in the form of a still layer between you and the environment. This is known as the "boundary layer," and its effectiveness is demonstrated most powerfully by penguins, the most cold-adapted animal in the world. Penguins are able to keep their core temperature at 98.6°F (37°C) when the Antarctic environment is -40°F (-40°C), even before the cold continent's 90-mph winds are taken into account.

To maintain their boundary layer, penguins have 300 percent more feathers than any other bird. Then, despite gathering in huge groups, they barely touch one another to prevent their feathers from being squashed and risking the loss of this essential insulative layer of air around their bodies. Additionally, while humans can lose heat through blood flow to the muscles in their limbs, penguins have all of their muscles contained within their torsos.

Humans generally lose heat to the environment through two main mechanisms: evaporation and convection. Indoors, the boundary layer remains intact, so heat loss is minimal. When outside, however, the flow of air disrupts this insulative boundary layer—in fact, at a mere 9 mph—so we lose this layer completely and consequently cool much quicker.

Water evaporating from the skin is an extremely effective way to lose heat. This is why humans evolved to maintain our body temperature in hot environments through sweating. Unfortunately, for the exposed swimmer, evaporative heat loss from water clinging to the body also happens in the cold. So after a swim, when you are standing on the beach in the wind, you lose even more heat from the combined effect of the wind and wet due to increased evaporation.

Therefore, I recommend first drying off with a towel as quickly as possible, and then putting on sufficient clothes to keep that still layer of air next to the body and protect you from the windchill. When it's super-cold, I use two changing robes specially designed for outdoor swimmers. But you could also layer up with a wool base layer, hoodie, thick jacket, and a pair of sweatpants or other suitable combination. The (generally expensive) specialist kit is convenient but not necessary.

And before you get in, make sure to place this gear in a convenient place for a rapid exit.

After one of our Norwegian dips among the sea ice, my eleven-year-old son, Ib, observed what a luxury it was to put on warm clothes. Of course, the clothes weren't warm at all, but they felt warm relative to the cold water. It took us less than a minute to get dry and put on two layers of clothes before we started walking home—and that exercise warmed us up further. It's worth noting that the senses are often so numbed by the water that cold air doesn't feel that chilly. At least at first. But rest assured, the air is cold, and your body temperature will continue to fall after getting out of the water. So get warm and keep warm by moving fast.

A lot of gnarly old-timers, aghast at the recent rise in the number of cold water swimmers, are against wearing robes, but robes reduce heat loss and provide your body with protection from the wind. My only issue with them is that the most effective ones are bulky and heavy. This can be a problem if I need to carry them around with me all day afterward.

As for towels, any kind will do, but I'm a fan of lightweight microfiber towels. Even the biggest microfiber towels pack down so small that I can take them, along with a pair of goggles and trunks, almost anywhere in anticipation of the need for an emergency swim. And they help me maintain my not inconsiderable modesty.

Most swimmers get out of cold water feeling mostly warm inside, but due to a phenomenon known as "afterdrop," our core temperature may fall—and continue to fall—for more than thirty minutes after we've gotten out of the water.

This is a further example of how the second law of thermodynamics applies to outdoor swimming. Heat flows naturally from an object at a higher temperature to an object at a lower temperature, so following a dip, since our insides are warmer than our outsides, heat flows from our body's core to its periphery. This is why we need to prevent further loss of heat from our skin and move around or exercise to warm ourselves up.

The body is very clever, of course. The reason we shiver when we're cold is because all that involuntary muscular activity creates heat. Sometimes this is enough. But on colder days, or after a cold water swim, we need further heat input from more muscular activity. This is why I recommend exercising both before and after a swim. Be careful, however: If you feel dizzy after a swim, or while exercising, sit or lie on the floor straight away. Wrap yourself as warmly as possible and don't get up again until the feeling has passed

That said, while I prefer exercising to warm up postswim, there are other common, enjoyable, but not necessarily as effective methods, such as taking warm showers, drinking warm beverages, and getting into a sauna. Some people express concerns over hot showers and drinks, but I think these worries are a little misplaced. With a tiny bit of caution and common sense, there is no danger.

Showers have two potential problems. The one I hear most often is that they open up blood vessels in the skin too rapidly, which causes blood to rush out from the core and could lead to a drop in blood pressure and fainting. However, while a legitimate concern, in nearly two decades I've not come across it in real life.

HYPOTHERMIA

During a swim, it is important to distinguish between acclimating to the cold and signs that you are becoming hypothermic.

While challenging yourself to cold is rewarding, swimming to hypothermia is a tangible risk. Some studies show that any drop below our normal temperature range of 97.7 to 99.5°F, or 36.5 to 37.5°C, is associated with increased complications during and after surgery, although accidental hypothermia is defined by a core temperature of 95°F (35°C) or less. My own medical research and experience indicates that any drop below normal has a deleterious effect on comfort and function, and by the time the core temperature is officially hypothermic, things are really serious.

Hypothermia comes on gradually, and its symptoms include shivering, impaired coordination, sluggishness, weakness, and difficulty speaking due to jaw stiffness.

While everyone's body is different, and while every swim is different, here are the warning signs of hypothermia. Look out for these in yourself and in your fellow swimmers. A good way to remember them is to think of the "umbles":

Grumbles—negative mental outlook

Stumbles—has a stiff gait and a tendency to trip

Fumbles—slow reaction time, reduced coordination

Mumbles—an inability to enunciate words clearly

In reality, it is rare for people to become clinically and potentially harmfully hypothermic. During a cold water swim, our core temperature certainly lowers, but usually only slightly and not enough to cause significant problems or concerns. Occasionally, however, someone has just a little too much fun in the water or pushes themselves a little too far or too long. They may start to get the "umbles," and at first it can seem amusing. They laugh at their own inability to talk or walk without stumbling. But soon the umbles interfere with our ability to look after ourselves.

Thus, be mindful of the signs of hypothermia in everyone, including yourself. That's part of what it means to be a member of the friendly and helpful outdoor swimming community. We always care for our fellow swimmers. If someone looks like they need help, they do. Give them help and don't waste time.

Swimming with others is not just fun. It's about safety in the water.

A more likely danger from a hot shower is the potential for burning the skin. Because your skin has been numbed by the cold, you may not realize if the water is too hot or scalding. Also, because there's a lack of blood flow, that excess heat will not be carried away promptly and could accumulate and damage the skin. My advice is to start with a lukewarm shower and only turn the heat up as feeling comes back to your skin.

This mirrors what's done in hospitals. When patients with accidental hypothermia are treated, the aim is to warm them up at roughly the same rate they would have cooled down, which is a reasonable working principle.

Hot drinks are a source of concern due largely to the mistaken idea that your body will be fooled by the warmth in your stomach and think that it is no longer cold. Again, the thinking is that the blood vessels to the skin will open up and could cause you to faint.

In reality, the actual quantity of heat in a cup—whether it's hot chocolate, tea, or coffee—has next to zero effect on the body's temperature control system.

The most adverse effect I've witnessed is people shivering so much they couldn't hold their cups steady, which caused them to spill their drinks over themselves. In other words: While a warm drink is always welcome, reserve it for pleasure rather than a remedy.

Saunas, meanwhile, are great—and safe—both before and after swims. This is because the warmth comes from the air, which contains significantly less heat energy than water. Consider the difference between putting your hand in a 212°F (100°C) oven and putting your hand in a pot of boiling water. Millions of patients have been warmed before and after surgery by blowing warm air around them with—as long as the correct equipment is used— an almost zero rate of heat injury.

As you warm up after a cold water swim, remember to appreciate the moment when you feel completely transformed. One of my favorite things is to feel my body when I get out and mentally compare it to how it felt just a few short moments previously, before I got in. It may be that I now feel the wind and rain as a pleasurable sensation when, before, they were causing me so much discomfort that I was questioning my sanity. Or conversely, it may be the complete disappearance of the pain, stiffness, and generalized fatigue from the ten-mile cycle before my swim.

Leaving the water, take in the moment and all your physical sensations. They may be pleasurable, such as the caress of the wind on your cold skin, or not, such as the stones digging into your feet. Listen to the sound of waves crashing or the water lapping, the beating of your own heart, the laughter and cries of delight echoing all around you.

All these sensations connect us with the physical world. Nothing exists except in relation to other things—our senses, heightened by the challenge presented by the cold, form a powerful connection with the world and bring us back to life. At the same time, the inner transformation makes us feel that we can glide through space and time with ease, possessed with a new clarity of thought and a welcome lightness of mind and body.

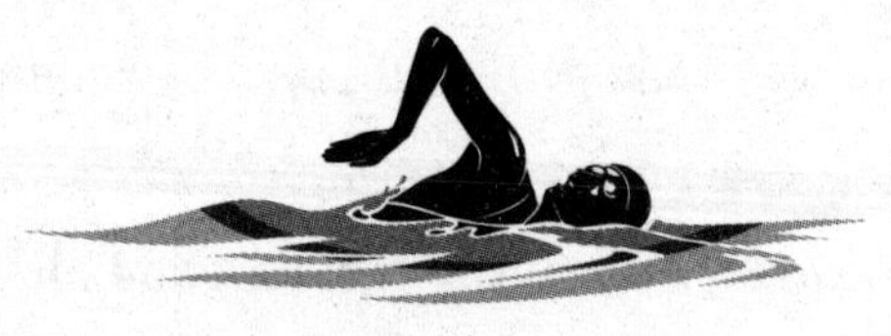

PART III

The Cold Water Swim Cure

CHAPTER 7

"RECOVER MYSELF IN THE SEA"

Chronic Pain

NOW IN HIS EARLY FIFTIES, Grant has suffered from chronic back pain since injuring his back surfing at age twenty. Up until then, he was incredibly active, playing squash and on his way to becoming a professional cyclist, although, he says, surfing was "his life." Though six feet tall (183 centimeters), he weighed just 140 pounds (63 kilograms). He enjoyed the perfect build for a cyclist or a squash player, but he was also ripe for a debilitating back injury.

One week before his twenty-first birthday, while surfing the waves off the Devon coast, his back "just went." The next morning, he woke up to find he couldn't move—an extremely frightening experience, especially for a young man. His muscles had gone into spasm. After his general practitioner dismissed his pain, Grant spent what little money he had on an MRI scan, which revealed that his L5-S1 intervertebral disc had completely blown out and was pressing onto his sciatic nerve. He underwent his first operation in September 1991.

Though his pain persisted, Grant managed to get back to surfing—although he had to give up cycling at a high level. To pursue his passion, he took a job as the manager of a holiday park to surf as much as he could. Nearly twenty years later, however, he blew out the same disc a second time, and in 2015, he blew out the disc above it.

This spelled the end of his surfing. Grant withdrew from his circle of friends and the community he had been part of for years because spending time on the same beaches he had enjoyed so much was now just too painful. This is when a vicious circle of pain and depression set in.

By the autumn of 2020, Grant was taking a cocktail of strong painkillers, including pregabalin (originally an anti-epileptic drug) and two powerful opioids, morphine sulphate and tramadol. This was despite having worked hard on developing routines that allowed him to lead as full a life as his condition would allow. Grant realized that he was dependent on these drugs and wanted to come off them. He tried going cold turkey but quickly found himself unable to cope with the withdrawal effects, which reminded him of a nasty hangover—headache, dizziness, body aches, and nausea. He also lacked energy and felt irritable and down. Unlike a hangover, however, the effects of his withdrawal lasted several weeks. He says, "I felt a genuine craving to start taking the pills again."

Still, Grant didn't just sit around feeling sorry for himself. He had a relatively active job as a painter and decorator. When he wasn't working, he spent hours walking along the water, beachcombing for treasure and trinkets, and collecting driftwood. The key to managing his pain, he figured out, was to keep moving. If he didn't, he couldn't move at all.

His ad hoc regimen proved so effective most people didn't have a clue he was suffering from chronic pain and depression. Like many stiff-upper-lip British men, he didn't want to be a burden or a whiner. Instead, he kept his pain and discomfort to himself, which only exacerbated his loneliness and alienation. "Dealing with mental health issues is a lonely business," he told me, shaking his head.

Thankfully, swimming provided relief. In the summer, he swam in the ocean, and when the weather turned cold, he took frequents dips in a local indoor pool. This wasn't enough to break the cycle of depression and pain, however. These grew so bad he nearly returned to his doctor to ask for another course of antidepressants. For the first time in his two decades of suffering, he also considered asking for a referral to a specialist pain clinic. Then by chance he saw a feature on his local BBC news about our first Chill Therapy course. Grant canceled his doctor's appointment and immediately signed up for some cold water swimming.

The course started in October, when the water was an unwelcoming 59°F (15°C). Shivering on the shore, Grant gingerly stepped into the surf. The shock of cold startled his senses awake, and he fought the instinct to retreat into his warm, cozy car. When he got home, he realized he was no longer in pain.

PAIN IS SIMPLE, PAIN IS COMPLEX

I work from basic principles, and admittedly, I struggle to remember facts. However, I do remember one definition from my postgraduate exams, the one for pain: "An unpleasant sensory and emotional experience associated with, or resembling that associated with, actual or potential tissue damage."

Pain is as simple as that. And not.

Everyone instinctively believes they understand the word *pain*. But when we stop to consider its meaning in full, it's quite extraordinary how one short word can translate into such an incredibly complex concept. So complex, in fact, the International Association for the Study of Pain (IASP) spent two years revising—or, rather, expanding upon—the accepted definition of pain to include six key characteristics.

Our intuitive understanding of the word *pain* is, broadly speaking, what physiologists call "nociception," the (relatively) straightforward process of a noxious stimulus causing a pain receptor to fire off a signal to the brain. The complexities arise because of the multilayered interpretation of that signal in the brain. This is why pain, according to the IASP, is always a personal experience influenced, to varying degrees, by specific biological, psychological, and social factors. Individuals learn the concept of pain through life experiences. Pain usually serves an effective and important adaptive role—its feedback is instrumental in how we learn to avoid danger. However, glitches in the multilayered interpretation system may set up abnormal circuits in the brain, which can have adverse effects on our ability to function and our social and psychological well-being.

The extent to which the perception of pain is not as simple as the stimulation of pain receptors sending signals to the brain becomes obvious when we consider all the different types of pain. We may first think of pain in terms of physical injury, such as cutting ourselves or stubbing a toe. So far, so simple.

But the sources of pain are many, and go well beyond obvious injuries: from broken bones to abdominal cramps, childbirth, period pains, tooth abscess, angina, arthritic joint pain, headache, a trapped nerve, high fever, and more. And what of the pain of a broken heart?

Then there are the different characteristics of pain: varying intensity, sharp, dull, constant, spasmodic, focused, diffuse, aching, burning.

Many things also influence the perception of pain. Quite apart from the obvious physical distinctions—most notably the location of an injury and the source or cause of it—there are genetics, our mood, the context (battlefield versus athletic field), our upbringing, cultural values, religious beliefs, previous experiences, and external reinforcement.

Pain can also be acute—such as when we stub a toe or immediately following an operation. Or chronic—such as when the initial stimulus is long gone and yet, years later, we are still suffering from its lingering effects. Acute pain is highly amenable to standard pharmacological interventions, that is, medicine. But chronic pain is thought to arise from the abnormal firing of neural circuits long after the adaptative function has passed.

When we consider all the different processes that underlie our subjective experience of pain, it becomes immediately apparent how incredibly diverse it is. Thus, it might seem a little odd that, for the most part, we treat all pain in the same way: with a limited number of medicines.

In 1986, the World Health Organization (WHO) published their "analgesic ladder" (recently updated in 2020), which forms the basis for the treatment of pain around the world. The first step of treatment focuses on paracetamol (acetaminophen) and anti-inflammatories like ibuprofen. Increasing in potency, the second step adds in the so-called "light" opioids, such as codeine, plus other nonopioids like gabapentin, an anti-epileptic drug. As you can see, there's not much of a leap to the third step, which recommends the use of morphine and stronger opioids. The invasive treatments in step four highlight procedures that target the nerves themselves.

This basic framework offers no specific mention of nonpharmacological interventions. The analgesic ladder also skips over the uncomfortable reality of side effects and a person's increased tolerance to medications, especially opioids. Codeine perfectly illustrates this issue. Although qualifying as a "light opioid," the only reason it has an effect is because the body converts around 10 percent into the "strong" opioid, morphine. In other words, the differentiation is cultural rather than pharmacological. However, 10 percent of the population cannot metabolize codeine, which robs them of the pain-relief benefits of morphine but, unfortunately, still exposes them to the side effects, including constipation and nausea. More problematic is the disturbing fact that 5 to 29 percent of the world's population are classified as ultra-rapid metabolizers. If they ingest codeine, it's possible that they end up "getting" dangerously high levels of morphine.

Unfortunately, the pharmacological means of treating pain are extremely limited, a troubling fact made only worse by the rising complaints of pain and the growing demand for relief around the world. In 2017, the US National Bureau of Economic Research published an article analyzing survey data from 2011. It showed that Americans reported aches and pains more often than any other nation. According to the survey, 34.1 percent of Americans reported feeling physical pain "often" or "very often." Australia was not too far behind, at 31.7 percent, closely followed by the United Kingdom, at 29.4 percent. All three nations enjoy advanced healthcare systems, with the United States spending, *per capita*, more than any other nation. With such a limited range of and perspective on treatment options for such a complex issue, however, such a high prevalence of pain is not entirely surprising.

The limited utility of drugs and the lack of perspective isn't the only problem. Another big issue is expectation. In their book *Ouch! Why Pain Hurts, and Why It Doesn't Have To*, authors Margee Kerr and Linda Rodriguez McRobbie argue convincingly that modern, Western culture has "a socially dysfunctional relationship with pain." This is due to many interlinked causes. First, there is the mechanical view of the body: If something's wrong with the body, we try to fix it in the same way we'd fix a car, by tinkering with or replacing parts. And just like how cars have become so filled with expensive technology and electronics that we often need specialists to repair them, we tend to believe only medical specialists can repair our failing bodies. This is exacerbated by advertising that makes us feel bad that we don't have the most up-to-date product. Ads for analgesics promote an image and expectation of a completely pain-free existence, which ignores the fact that "bearable" pain is not an unreasonable aim, or that the drugs themselves have side effects that are often worse than a moderate—and manageable—amount of pain. I'm forever pointing out to patients undergoing hernia repair that the pain from the constipation caused by the codeine they are inevitably prescribed is likely to be far worse than any analgesic effect codeine will have on their symptoms.

Nearly forty years ago, Harvard psychiatrist Arthur Barsky provided data showing that the United States was becoming more sensitive to pain. He highlighted community surveys from the 1920s, which found respondents had 0.82 episodes of serious illness a year. He then contrasted this statistic with numbers from the 1980s, when these episodes increased to 2.12 per year. Though people were objectively healthier, they believed they felt worse. They suffered more pain, more frequently.

There are many possible reasons for this increasing sensitivity. Altered expectations is one. Another is a greater prevalence of depression. The relationship between depression and pain also highlights the problems caused by an emphasis on analgesic medication. People who are depressed show abnormalities in the body's release of its own endogenous opioid chemicals. As a result, opioids are less effective at treating their pain. Second, depression tends to exacerbate and prolong pain, which interferes with postoperative recovery. Mark Sullivan, a professor of psychiatry at the University of Washington, has a theory. "Depressed people," he argues, "are in a state of alarm. They're fearful, or frozen in place. There's a heightened sense of threat."

This heightened sense of threat heightens the sensation of pain.

Pain is, ultimately, a construct of the mind. Therefore, when we consider its treatment and effects, we need to understand its perception as well as its actual cause. Many types of pain have a physical basis that can be treated by correcting the underlying injury—such as a broken bone—and ameliorated with painkillers. However, our treatments for pain will be more effective if we consider the many factors that influence a person's perception of pain rather than concentrating only on a physical source. Pain arises from the interaction of our body and our mind.

Furthermore, our perception of pain can be modified by nonpharmacological means. This can be as simple as the color of the tablets we swallow. A couple of fascinating studies back up this claim. One showed that, following dental surgery, 79 percent of patients had adequate pain relief with red tablets, as opposed to just 73 percent with white tablets. Another study, which looked at the efficacy of different colored tablets and colored placebos in patients with rheumatoid arthritis, found that the red placebo was as effective as the best active drug. Blue and green placebos, however, were described by patients as average.

Another straightforward approach is to reframe our experience of pain so that we regard it as positive. For example, in a sports or training context, it's common to hear the phrase, "no pain, no gain." With good reason. Postoperatively, doctors sometimes reframe pain as "a sign that your body is healing." Indeed, a 2013 study found that when the meaning of a painful experience was reframed from detrimental to beneficial, participants exhibited a much higher tolerance. Even more interesting, this increased tolerance seemed to have been aided by the activation of the body's own opioid and cannabinoid systems. It is much better to have the body control its own in-built analgesic system because this helps prevent the development of resistance to drugs—and thus the need for increasing dosages to achieve the same effect—and their side effects.

On the other hand, external reinforcement can adversely reframe our experience of pain. One of my pet gripes is when, after first waking up following surgery, patients are asked, "How much pain do you have?" Asking someone to focus on their pain is only going to highlight any discomfort and may even impede the healing process. In my opinion, I prefer asking a more "functional" question, such as "Is the pain bearable or not?" Since the experience of pain is subjective, it's more useful to focus on qualitative distinctions rather than quantitative ones.

It's in our best interest—and best for our health—to let pain serve its adaptive role where appropriate: to help us get better and gain more control of how we feel.

COLD WATER SWIMMING: A NEW APPROACH TO MANAGING PAIN

On the surface, it may seem that getting into cold water for pain and symptom relief is contradictory. It's like treating pain with pain. When we look at it more closely, however, it isn't illogical at all. First, the pain from cold water swimming is reframed as beneficial—participants know that it has been shown to be an effective intervention and their own experience of swimming is that it fosters the feeling of well-being and, hopefully, symptom relief.

Until someone tries it, though, this doesn't seem self-evident. During a live BBC radio interview, I explained that, while it is painful getting into cold water, you feel so good for the rest of the day, and the interviewer closed by commenting that you also feel better when you stop hitting your head against a brick wall. While funny, this teasing remark misses the crucial difference between the pain of cold immersion and of physical injury. If you batter your forehead against a brick wall, you're still going to feel pain after you stop due to the resulting physical damage—contusions, cuts, and likely concussion symptoms. Only positive repercussions follow a quick dip in cold waters.

Being able to get in and out of the water and overcoming the initial discomfort develops resilience. This reduces the sensitivity to a threat, and many medical professionals now say this sensitivity contributes to pain. A review of pain in orthopedics found that a focus on patient "self-efficacy"—that is, when patients take control of their own treatment process—in arthritic knee care and physical activity was beneficial. It also confirmed that physical activity and exercise during the rehabilitation period after total knee arthroplasty can improve global function, benefit other joints with osteoarthritis, and help maintain global health.

Another often overlooked side effect of surgery is something called "neuropathic pain," or when pain persists though there isn't any apparent damage to a nerve or body part. Neuropathic pain is an extremely difficult condition to treat, and it can arise without any apparent cause. However, I read about one case where a patient had this condition following a chest operation. Afterward, he coincidentally took up open water swimming and was pleasantly surprised to find that it led to a complete resolution of his symptoms.

While one experience is not sufficient to recommend anything as a universal treatment, it does add further support to the contention that cold water swimming can be an effective activity in a multifaceted approach to the management of the multifaceted problem of pain.

And there are signs that perceptions are changing. Susie, one of my anaesthetic colleagues, was delighted to relate to me the reply from one of the medical students she was teaching. When asked what alternative treatments exist for pain, one medical student suggested cold water swimming. These are the doctors of tomorrow.

"THE CHILL POOL IS MY TRAMADOL": GRANT'S COLD WATER SWIM CURE

Cold water swimming isn't a panacea that gets rid of all pain, but it clearly has some kind of analgesic effect. It provides the movement and exercise that help specific and global function. As Grant experienced, it also can provide company and a positive distraction that can make lingering, chronic pain more bearable.

An hour after Grant got home following his first session, he realized he was pain-free. This reinforces the hypothesis that pain is more in the brain than the body—Grant's back must have still been sending the same pain signals, yet his brain was processing them in a different way.

When asked what alternative treatments exist for pain, one medical student suggested cold water swimming. These are the doctors of tomorrow.

No one has yet done studies to show how this works, but my working theory is that the intensity of the cold stimulus in some way reboots the neural circuits, reframing and rewiring them to function more appropriately.

Still today, Grant remains pain-free for about thirty minutes to an hour after a swim, and the discomfort remains at a lower level for the rest of the day. In late 2021, Grant was thrilled to pass his first "chilliversary," and he says that cold water swimming is "the best coping mechanism I have developed to cope with my chronic back pain. All the benefits are still there, and I'm happy to say I remain off the opioid painkillers." He still suffers, but the only medication he takes is an occasional pregabalin capsule, which helps treat his neuropathic pain.

Grant's "head space" feels better, too. While he partly attributes this to the cold water, he credits a number of other factors as well. He emphasizes the significance of starting out with an organized group. Knowing that there are lifeguards, as well as experienced instructors, makes it possible for him to enjoy swimming without having to worry about safety. Everyone motivates one another. Grant describes pulling into the parking lot as "brutal" sometimes. Like me, he often asks himself, *What am I doing here?* Then he reminds himself why, and it all clicks into place. Everything makes sense. In fact, in the beginning, as autumn turned to winter and the water got colder, he started to "feel the bite and enjoy it even more. . . . The cold makes it more intense and accelerates things." He loves to look at his cold water swimming partners before they get in—the look of apprehension, the struggle to find the courage to take the plunge—and then compare their faces after the swim, when everyone is laughing, their chests puffed out in exhilaration and pride. It seems to him that they come out surrounded by a warm, orange glow that reminds him of the British TV commercials from the seventies and eighties for Ready Brek hot cereal, whose tagline was "central heating for kids."

In addition to alleviating his chronic pain, which transformed him, Grant's cold water swimming reoriented his worldview and his years-long misperception of how his pain has limited him. He is once again immersed in nature, which is a key part of his identity that he believed he had sacrificed for good because of his pain. He's also made a few stalwart friends in the process.

What Grant loves about the nature of the community is that it's noncompetitive and feels "tribal." He's part of a tribe that's a little bit out there—just like he was in his surfing days. Whenever he goes looking for other swimming spots, he finds more people with the same idea. And while he loves the rough-and-tumble energy of the ocean, he finds tranquillity in a favorite freshwater pond, where the experience is heightened by the birds and the peace and quiet. "The chill pool is my tramadol," he says.

"I FEEL I CAN LET GO": DAVID'S COLD WATER SWIM CURE

While the joys and benefits of the cold are something new for Grant, David is one of the few people I know who's been swimming outdoors longer than me, and his connections go back even further.

David is the link to the whole history of the Brighton Swimming Club, the oldest swimming club in England. His grandmother's grandfather, George Brown, was one of the founding members back in 1860 when sea swimming was the only option.

Interestingly, his early experiences of swimming were somewhat inauspicious. "I failed to learn to swim through the compulsory classes held for junior school children in Brighton's North Road Baths," he recalls, referencing the Victorian buildings he swam in—or rather didn't swim in—during the 1940s. "What I did gain was fearlessness in the water. I could happily sit on the bottom watching my classmates' legs."

The building featured a thirty-six-yard swimming pool, but it also provided "slipper" baths for people who didn't have a bathtub at home. A quarter of a century later, I too learned how to swim in these baths, and to this day I can still feel the bitter and breathtaking cold of that water.

David's ongoing connection with the ocean began shortly after his failed swim lessons, when he discovered that seawater supported his body better than freshwater. "I can recall to this day the sensation of flying in the sea beneath the water after establishing control of my body and breathing amid the waters. It was an experience deeply imprinted on me."

As much as he enjoyed swimming, the activity very much went on the back burner over the next few years. "Sea swimming was forgotten except as a social activity and as a break from being a bingo caller on the pier as a holiday job," he admits. David subsequently moved on to be the art director at a minor public school, where he taught alongside his wife, running the school's adventure training. "I ended up using the cliff and rock falls, not swimming, for I had found pupils could not cope with the cold water of the sea."

David realized that he was burnt out in his job when he noticed he was becoming as irascible as his own former teachers. When he delved deeper, he found that "difficulties with my teaching turned out to rest on a solution to the body-mind problem. To escape the struggle with words, I went back to sea swimming. Being in the sea involves body and mind. The current has to be felt in order to determine the appropriate vector to swim along in order to reach a targeted area."

Initially, David swam on his own, but members of the Brighton Swimming Club eventually invited David to swim with them through the winter. "I swam long distances and experienced the magic of catching the tide when it first flowed back along the River Cuckmere. I once swam so far I joined a school of bass. Their freedom with water was mine."

When he turned fifty, however, David was, he says, "gifted with osteoarthritis" in his left big toe. On its own, this might not have been so bad, but osteoarthritis also "crept up" through his body and into his neck, which "robbed me of my breaststroke." He had to devise a novel stroke, using paddles and fins. "I was fifty-eight when arthritis finally overtook me. It was a truly depressing state of affairs. Without flippers and hand paddles, I would be lost."

Despite his increasing physical disability, David kept coming up with new ways to engage with the ocean. Thinking back to his experience swimming with the bass, he says, "I could not let the fish be once I saw their presence and had to devise a means of catching them. Making and shaping is something I love doing."

As a teacher, David created "adventures" for his pupils. One involved having them improvise a beach shelter using a plastic sheet, some plywood, and rope. Once finished, students cooked sausages as a well-earned reward—using water that flowed from the cliff and driftwood to provide fuel. Channeling this spirit, David devised an aquatic activity he calls "swishing," a combination of swimming and fishing. He attaches mackerel hooks to a homemade bamboo rod and lets the line trail behind him as he swims through the water with fins on his feet, which lets him keep a steady pace. The most difficult (and perhaps distracting) part is removing the fish from the hook and transferring it into the net bag—all while floating in the sea. This is another example of sea swimming involving both body and mind.

Arthritis literally means "inflammation of the joints." This extraordinarily general term could be applied to something as simple as the pain in one's knees after a long walk. However, it usually refers to either osteoarthritis or rheumatoid arthritis. Both involve degeneration of the joints. The most common form is osteoarthritis, in which the cartilage that caps the bones in the joints is worn away, and it is usually related to wear and tear, old injuries, and being overweight. It can also run in families.

The disease results in an increase in the water content of cartilage and a reduction in the strong, protein component. This structural imbalance means the cartilage steadily degenerates and also impairs the body's ability to repair itself. The process can be exacerbated by unhealthy levels of inflammatory molecules in the system, which increase with the pain as bone rubs on bone.

One of the mainstays of treatment is anti-inflammatory drugs. As with all drugs, anti-inflammatories have unwanted side effects, including stomach ulcers. Regular cold water swimming, on the other hand, can reduce inflammation in a more natural and controlled manner—most immediately through the direct stimulation of the parasympathetic nervous system and, over the long term, through adaptation.

Our research team was not, therefore, surprised that in our 2019 survey of people already using cold water swimming as a form of self-treatment, musculoskeletal conditions were the second-largest group after mental health. Of our 722 respondents, 21 percent said they experienced some form of musculoskeletal pain and 83 percent reported some level of improvement following a session of cold water swimming.

To get by, David now needs a cocktail of painkillers, including opioids. Even going for short journeys to the hospital—or a quick visit to some of his favorite swimming spots—is difficult. He tells me, "Opioids provide a platform, squashing pain enough to allow writing and reading. . . . They get me down to the seafront, even though sometimes the struggle becomes daunting. But by thinking of the gain awaiting, I keep going. If I misjudge the weather, and the sea is too big for me to manage, getting home is a daunting task."

David has tried other nonpharmacological ways of dealing with his condition and the pain, including many strange diets and the vinegar cure, but they were "no help."

"Physiotherapists have tried to assist me several times. Their efforts were counterproductive." During one hospital stay, he tried to come off "the poison I consider the opioids." However, despite his determination, any "movement almost had me screaming."

The only time David's pain levels are reduced to a level at which he can function is during and after his daily swim. While it is known that the symptoms of osteoarthritis often improve with movement, cold water swimming also seems to have an additional analgesic effect. In our 2019 survey, 79 percent of people with neurological problems, which includes chronic pain, reported an improvement. This may be as a result of the support the water provides for the body, especially higher-density saltwater, and of "distraction," due to the need to concentrate on the prevailing conditions. For this reason, according to David, the "calm placid seas are less welcome than crisply boisterous ones or seas that make my heart leap and call into doubt my calculations of safety." He also gives partial credit to being in the sea at dawn. He says, "The sight of the sun emerging from the water is eye-catching and stands to reveal the direction in which the Earth is turning . . . and the endless horizon."

Following his morning swim, David reports a welcome period of four to six hours when his symptoms are reduced. When you see him cantering up the beach with his crutch, as I often do, you would find it hard to believe that, come the afternoon, he finds it difficult to get out of a chair.

Over time, the disease process has caused his hip joints to disintegrate, despite the fact his bones in general are, as his surgeon told me, like those of a forty-year-old. As a result, he is unable to "readily raise myself if knocked down. Pushing down on the shingle with arms stiff, wiggling my bum back away from the sea, I realize my loss of mobility."

Despite this, the ocean still provides a lifeline—both by providing some respite from his chronic pain and allowing David to actively "live," at least for a few hours every day. He says, if there's one thing he wants to pass on from telling his story, it is to "wake people up to the responsibility for 'being' on which 'well-being' can be taken to rest."

He continues:

> It was by literally seeming to "recover myself" in the sea—able to be an exploiter of its tumult, not a victim—that the benefit or contribution to pain relief and well-being offered by the ocean became apparent. Nothing equated with the challenge of the deep.

Obviously as I age, muscular power diminishes, and cold appears more of a deterrent, but the relief I get being able to move and the illusion of freedom is enough. I feel I can let go, knowing I can snort out water that floods over my face, hang on long enough beneath the waves to get myself to safety, albeit farther out to sea, and wait for a lull. There can be nothing more satisfying than knowing I can paddle along beneath the canopy of the sky, always long enough to escape feeling confined by my body or imprisoned by thoughts and beliefs I still haven't taken responsibility for.

CHAPTER 8

"IT JUST FEELS LIKE HEAVEN"

Migraines

IN A DARKENED BEDROOM, A YOUNG WOMAN SUFFERS quietly under a striped comforter, her right hand gently cradling her forehead as if it were an egg. "My head really hurts," Beth says into the camera, which holds her face tightly in frame. "It hurts, like in my head. I started to notice that my vision started to go funny and then it got tingly around this eye and my lip. And now my head hurts a lot."

This is an opening scene from the 2020 documentary *100 Days of Vitamin Sea,* which chronicles Beth's attempt to retake control of her health and restore joy in her life through cold water swimming. A native of North Wales, Beth had been experiencing migraines, on and off, for more than sixteen years, ever since she was nine, but in July 2017, she was diagnosed with "chronic migraine." At that point, she was averaging twenty-eight migraine days a month.

Chronic migraine is a neurological disease, defined as episodic headaches that last anywhere from four to seventy-two hours, at least fifteen times a month. To classify as a migraine, it must come with two of the following symptoms: unilateral pain, throbbing, and aggravation on movement; pain of moderate or severe intensity accompanied with nausea or vomiting; or exquisite sensitivity to light or sounds.

In the United States and Western Europe, more than one in ten adults—and one in five women, for whom the condition is around three times as common—will suffer a migraine attack during the year. And a tenth of these sufferers—approximately 2.5 million people in North America alone—suffer weekly attacks.

A day with severe migraine is as disabling as a day with quadriplegia, and according to the WHO Global Burden of Disease report, migraines rank alongside psychosis and dementia as the most disabling chronic conditions. However, in terms of its burden on individuals and society, a migraine has the dubious distinction of affecting the young and being incredibly common.

Typical attacks consist of four phases, although not all may be present for any given attack: the prodrome, the aura, the attack, and the postdrome.

The prodrome occurs one or two days before a migraine. It includes subtle physiological changes, including constipation, mood swings that range from depression to euphoria, sudden cravings for food, neck stiffness, increased thirst and urination, and frequent yawning.

The aura arrives with visual disturbances, such as flashes of light or blind spots, and perhaps other sensations, such as tingling on one side of the face or in an arm or leg, uncontrollable jerking or other movements, and difficulty speaking.

The attack itself can last hours or days. "Sometimes," Beth says, "they just hit you in the head for, like, forty hours." Attacks have such a profound effect on people's lives that, rather than measure the actual symptoms, the severity of the condition is most usefully assessed by marking the time lost as a result.

Following an attack, the postdrome leaves a person feeling drained, confused, and washed out for up to a day, although some people do report feeling a period of elation. Sudden head movement might bring on the pain again briefly.

In Beth's case, the four phases of a typical migraine attack forced her to put off her PhD program in marine biology, even though she tried every available treatment protocol, from intravenous opioids to Botox injections. Nothing seemed to reduce the frequency and intensity of her attacks. Nor did they offer her a way to continue any of the day-to-day things we all consider a normal part of life. A neurologist, in a typically despairing appointment, told her the best she could hope for was limiting her migraines to four per week. At least until she got older, he told her, when she started going through menopause. "I am twenty-five years old," she recalls in the film, "and my doctor is saying don't worry it will get better in twenty-five years." Chronic migraine runs in families. In Beth's case, migraines can be traced back through five generations of women, starting with her great-great-grandmother, who was born in 1887. Although she didn't know what it was at the time, Beth's grandmother, Merle, had her first migraine headache at nine years old. As Merle recounts in the film, they "didn't know much about it then, and they don't know much about it now, do they?" Her doctors dismissed her migraines as minor headaches. They told her to take a tablet, shut up, and stop moaning. To get through an attack, Merle hummed to herself, believing that, if she didn't, she would die.

During an assembly, Merle experienced a particularly brutal migraine attack. "I thought, 'I can't see. I can't see the teacher. I can see the top of her head and her feet, but I can't see the middle. I can't hold the hymn book in my hand.' That fell to the floor."

At the end of assembly, she tried to explain to her teacher what was happening to her. All she could say was, "I've got a hardache." The teacher thought she was being insolent for not saying "headache," so she made her sit in the corridor for four hours until she was finally allowed to go home. Initially, Merle's doctor thought she might have meningitis. He diagnosed her migraines a few days later, after he looked it up in his medical books. Such was the level of ignorance.

Years later, her own daughter, Beth's mother, Jayne, came downstairs and said something that still breaks her heart. "Mum," Jayne said, "I've got a hardache."

Unfortunately, the severity of the condition has worsened through the generations.

Beth's migraines can force her to stay in her house, usually in bed under the covers, because of the pain radiating from her head through her body. "I've been having a migraine for seventeen minutes now," she continues in the film, "and it's like a big chunk of my vision on this side is just kind of gone—kind of blurred out and totally out of focus. I've got little black dots floating around. I feel all weak, and kind of dizzy, and not with it all. The pain started really quickly this time. It just hurts so much. It spreads out and it hurts in all my teeth like they might fall out, and it feels like my jaw is getting smaller. It's just so painful. So painful. And it's kind of scary too because you can't really think properly. I'm struggling even to think. The pain of it is just getting worse and worse, and there's pain in the back of my neck. It's a horrible feeling. There's just nothing you can do. Your head's just going to split open and you're going to die."

THE VITAMIN SEA

In 2017, Beth felt like her life was slipping away. At that point, she and her then-boyfriend, now-husband, Andy, decided to swim in the ocean for a hundred days in a row, over the winter of 2017–18, just to see what happened.

"I read that physical activity in nature was known to aid people with a variety of health conditions," Beth says in the film. "We both get so much of our energy from being in nature, but coming to terms with chronic illness, I lost touch with nature, and we lost touch with a part of our identity. We decided to embark on a challenge to swim in the sea in North Wales to learn more about where we live, to reconnect with nature, and to see how it makes us feel. We aren't expecting this to be cured, but we want to see if it can give us some peace."

Since Andy is also a filmmaker, they decided to chronicle their aquatic adventures as a side project. The resulting documentary, *100 Days of Vitamin Sea,* is a beautiful, emotional, and insightful exploration of Beth's health and wellness transformation.

In 2009, Professor Michael Depledge and Dr. William Bird proposed a notion called the "blue gym," which uses the ocean as a motivation for people to exercise outdoors. They have found that regular contact with natural environments provides three major health benefits: It reduces stress, increases physical activity, and creates stronger communities.

Other studies and my own findings support this. In our 2019 outdoor swimming survey, thirty-six people self-reported suffering from headaches or migraines. Of these, 94 percent found cold water swimming had a positive effect. Many explained that, following their cold water swims, their symptoms had greatly reduced, both in frequency and intensity. They also said it helped them reduce medication dependence. In case after case, cold water swimming seems to promote improved mental and physical health, while more rigorous studies indicate that it leads to life-changing experiences of reorientation, transformation, and connection—all of which Beth experienced.

Beth and Andy are hardly the first artists to chronicle their migraine experiences and symptoms. Way back in 3000 BCE, Mesopotamian poets translated their auras into verse, and a couple of millennia later, in 400 BCE, Hippocrates penned the following account of a patient's migraines: "He seemed to see something shining before him like a light, after a moment, a violent pain supervened in the right temple, then in all the head. Vomiting, when it became possible, was able to divert the pain and render it more moderate."

Though she never thought it might actually improve her symptoms, Beth found that swimming in the ocean provided a degree of immediate relief and also appeared to stall the effects of oncoming migraines. She also noted an overall reduction in the frequency and intensity of her migraine episodes.

Despite being so widespread and having such an impact on sufferers (not to mention its cost to society), very little is understood about the mechanisms underlying migraine.

During the aura, there is a change in electrical activity, which Andrew J. Whalen, a postdoctoral scholar at Penn State's Center for Neural Engineering, describes as "a rolling blackout, a chain reaction that moves across the brain causing swelling." In experimental models, this spreading depolarization can be prevented from developing through the application of a positive electrical charge.

When we immerse ourselves in cold water, a huge number of different nerves start firing. This sends a massive wave of electrical impulses to the brain, which may provide a positive electrical charge that can prevent the spreading depolarization experienced during the aura. This could explain Beth's observation that the frequency of her attacks reduced, since the sea was snuffing them out before they could take hold.

However, changes in electrical activity are not associated with other parts of the migraine. While the underlying mechanisms for these have remained uncertain, a recent discovery may have finally provided a breakthrough, while also clarifying how cold water swimming might help sufferers like Beth.

Researchers have discovered that the release of a neurotransmitter, with the particularly catchy name calcitonin gene-related peptide (CGRP for short), is associated with migraine attacks. This discovery has since led to the development of a new class of drugs—called more catchily "gepants"—that block this neurotransmitter, along with monoclonal antibodies. These drugs have been life-changing for some sufferers.

One of the theories about the underlying process at a cellular level is that CGRP causes neurogenic neuroinflammation—substances released by nerves in the brain that cause inflammation in the brain—which may be alleviated when the parasympathetic nervous system is stimulated. As I explain in chapter 4 ("Chill Out: Embrace the Cool to Stay Cool," page 76), parasympathetic stimulation occurs when we put our face in cold water, which might explain why cold water swimming has a similar positive effect to the new gepants drugs.

When we immerse ourselves in
cold water, a huge number of
different nerves start firing.

In 2021, the incredible work of the four doctors who were most instrumental in bringing gepants to clinical use won the Brain Prize, the highest award in neuroscience. However, we don't yet know if these medicines will work for everybody, and they are not universally available. In the meantime, approaches like cold water swimming can help people suffering from migraines manage their condition and regain some control of their lives in the process. Without a doubt, we have more to learn. Migraines involve complex neural interactions, and CGRP is only one of many different neurotransmitters that might be involved.

"THE PAIN JUST WASHES AWAY": BETH'S COLD WATER SWIM CURE

For Beth, during her one hundred days of swimming, it often took an extreme exercise of willpower to get out of the house and down to the beach: "You just can't wish yourself well. You have to be so proactive, but it's so difficult if you're in so much pain. The last thing you want to do is go down and stick your head in water that is eight degrees Celsius. We always love it, but it is hard to get in."

This difficulty is brilliantly captured in one powerful sequence during the film. Beth struggles down the beach very tentatively. Once in the water, though, she exclaims, "It just feels like heaven. God, I just feel so much better. It isn't a miracle cure. I can't explain it, but whatever it is I don't care. It's working. I just got me some free morphine, in the sea. The pain goes from a nine to a four. The pain just washes away. I'm still scared and panicked. But I wanted to die, and I couldn't cope with it, and now I feel like I can breathe."

Afterward, she reflects, "I had an absolutely killer migraine today, and I had to drag myself to the beach, but here never ever fails. I come into the sea just knowing I'm taking that step, putting one foot in front of the other, and trying my damned hardest is just enough some days. It's the most incredible empowering thing I've ever done."

At times, her symptoms were so bad, Beth wasn't able to make it to the beach, and so she tried the next best alternative, a cold bath. At one point in the film, she is crying, saying, "I'm really bloody suffering. I can't get out of the house."

Then, as she lowers herself into the bath, she says, "This hurts so much. But it's really helping."

Beth celebrates her experience as "the morphine-like analgesia of cold water." She says, "It isn't about fixing things. It's about making it easier to live with so that you can enjoy the journey of life despite the challenges that you are facing or lie ahead of you."

Andy agrees, and says in the film, "Beth's been battling a rift in space time that happens inside her brain. That's my theory on how migraines work anyway." What kind of medicine is going to be able to fix that?

Through sharing their story on social media, radio, and television, Beth and Andrew have brought support and help to many other chronic migraine sufferers. In the film, two people articulate what a difference swimming in the cold has made to them. Glynis says, "Boy, oh boy, has it changed my life. I would advise anyone to try it—it has had the most profound effect on my body."

Another woman named Beth wonderfully describes the experience: "You just feel weightless, and your worries and pain just melt away. It's not like the pain just goes away—you're still aware that the pain is still there—but it's not all-consuming. It's just like in the same way you have arms or legs. To me, when I'm in the water, I just feel so good. It's just like everything melts away."

At the end of the film, Beth emphasizes the importance of community in managing her condition: "As well as the loving support of our family and friends, we found huge support connecting with other migraineurs through social media; being part of a community of people trying to help each other get through a chronic illness. Everyone is just lifting each other up. We're a tribe."

CHAPTER 9

"ALERT, ALIVE, AND A SENSE OF EUPHORIA AND ACHIEVEMENT"

Fibromyalgia

THE TERM *FIBROMYALGIA* is really just a latinization of the words for fibrous tissues like tendons and ligaments (*fibro*) and muscular pain (*myalgia*). While chronic, widespread joint and muscular pain and diffuse aching or burning are a universal part of the diagnosis, people with the condition also suffer from a number of other problems.

Patients suffer from depression, anxiety, and fatigue—which can range from feeling tired to the debilitating exhaustion of a flu-like illness—as well as cognitive dysfunction, most notably a lack of concentration, temporary memory impairment, mixing words up, clumsiness, and dizziness. All of these symptoms contribute to a vicious circle of restless and entirely unrefreshing sleep. People with fibromyalgia wake up tired and stiff, often suffering from headaches, irritable bowels, and an acute sensitivity to changes in the weather, noise, bright lights, smoke, and other environmental factors.

People with mild to moderate cases of fibromyalgia are, with the right treatment, usually able to live a normal life. If symptoms are severe, however, people may not be able to hold down a paying job or be able to have an active social life. Between 2 and 5 percent of the population worldwide suffers from it.

While the condition sometimes develops without an obvious trigger, its onset is often associated with a trauma of some kind—anything from suffering a bad fall or surviving a car accident to contracting a viral infection or experiencing a life-altering, emotional event. The working theory is that fibromyalgia is the product of the brain's sudden, disordered processing of sensory information. That is, the wires in the brain and the body keep getting crossed. Brain scans of patients with fibromyalgia reveal a simultaneous increase in activation and a reduction in specific neurotransmitters, creating an imbalance that is debilitating. Disordered processing in the visual circuits and pain perception exacerbates the symptoms.

It should come as no surprise, then, that treating this complex jungle of cross-wired neural circuits is extremely difficult. While some medications work for some people, they don't work for others. Often, treating fibromyalgia requires patients to use drugs "off label," or for symptoms the drugs aren't licensed to treat. Such medications, older antidepressants in particular, provide only limited relief of discrete symptoms rather than actually treating the condition itself. Even at lower doses, these medications can have significant side effects.

What is really needed is some way to break this cycle and rewire the circuits.

RESETTING THOSE PESKY, CROSS-WIRED NEURAL CIRCUITS

One approach is cognitive behavioral training, which has been shown to be an effective and actionable therapeutic. This technique involves modifying a person's response to pain, changing behavior, and managing thoughts and emotions through cognitive restructuring, pain coping strategies, relaxation, and imagery techniques. This empowers people suffering from fibromyalgia to take more control of its myriad symptoms.

Dr. Mark Pellegrino is the medical director for rehabilitation at an Ohio hospital, and he specializes in the condition. He also suffers from fibromyalgia. He understands better than most physicians how difficult it is to make this switch in mindset and find the delicate balance of rest and activity that helps people stay on top of their condition—what he has described as an "exercise dilemma." Because the muscles are so tight and painful, they are often aggravated by any attempt to exercise. However, if the muscles aren't used enough, they can more easily flare up during any activity.

"Many people with fibromyalgia have had negative experiences with exercising," Dr. Pellegrino writes on the Fibromyalgia Action UK website. "The goal is to make exercise a positive experience for someone with fibromyalgia."

The best way to solve this dilemma, he says, is for people with fibromyalgia to participate in a light conditioning program, starting with a proper warm-up and followed by sustainable breathing techniques, proper posture, and an increased awareness of the body's response to activity—all of which are core components of Chill Therapy courses.

Indeed, a few people suffering from fibromyalgia have reported that cold water swimming eases their symptoms. As with chronic pain, perhaps the physical and emotional shock of the cold triggers a resetting of those pesky, cross-wired neural circuits, in much the same way cognitive behavioral therapy resets them through a psychological process.

Interestingly, there is an additional way in which cold water swimming may help. In 2021, scientists at King's College London published a paper in the *Journal of Clinical Investigation* hypothesizing that fibromyalgia may be caused by an autoimmune response that triggers the body's response to pain. This theory is in stark contrast to the prevailing wisdom that the condition's abnormal pain response arises entirely from the brain.

In their study, scientists harvested the blood from forty-four people with fibromyalgia and injected purified antibodies from it into mice. Immediately, the mice injected with the blood became more sensitive to pressure and cold, and they exhibited decreased strength and dexterity, particularly in their ability to grip objects with their paws. (Conversely, other mice were injected with antibodies from healthy people, and they were unaffected.) The affected mice recovered once the antibodies were flushed from their systems, which suggests that therapies like plasma exchange, which are designed to reduce antibody levels in patients with other autoimmune disorders, may be effective in fibromyalgia patients. But plasma exchange is a risky, complicated, and expensive procedure.

Autoimmune disorders are the result of an overzealous immune response in which, in essence, the body begins to attack itself. These attacks are characterized by inappropriately high levels of inflammation. Because cold water adaptation reduces levels of inflammation, that could be why it attenuates the symptoms of fibromyalgia, in much the same way cold water swimming benefits other autoimmune conditions, including inflammatory bowel disease and arthritis.

Perhaps cold water swimming won't cure fibromyalgia, but in two ways—through dampening an overenthusiastic immune system and providing an electrical reboot—it seems to have the potential to deliver real benefits. This is backed up by our Chill Therapy courses and surveys—coupled with anecdotal stories from other people with fibromyalgia—which show that it can alleviate the condition's most uncomfortable flare-ups over short and long periods of time.

Most people, of course, don't really care why something works. If a practice brings a much-needed respite from pain and discomfort, as well as relief from anxiety and negativity, then people willingly embrace it. This includes people like Laura Sanderson, Nikki Marshall, and Martin, a Chill Therapy alumnus.

"REVVED UP AND EXHILARATED FOR DAYS": LAURA, NIKKI, MARTIN, AND THE COLD WATER SWIM CURE

When Laura Sanderson was diagnosed with fibromyalgia, her doctor suggested she take cold water showers, but she wanted to get out and stretch her limits and her imagination. She started to swim in local spots in her native Wales, then over time, she swam throughout the United Kingdom.

She chronicled her efforts in a gorgeous and inspiring short documentary film, appropriately called *Hydrotherapy* (see Fin and Jack Davies in "Further Reading and Resources" for a YouTube link).

"Some days, I would feel one hundred years old," she recounts in the documentary. "I wouldn't be able to get out of bed. All of my muscles would ache and be painful to the touch, and on occasion, my joints would swell up. I started to swim outside, and the release in my muscles and joints was immediate, and I felt my body could flow freely."

Seeking out different types of water—"lakes, rivers, waterfalls"—she was able to minimize her pain, connect to the present moment, and experience only the immediate shock of the water, which she says restored her relationship with her body and with nature.

"Swimming on my own was a release, and it was the only time I could process and connect to the moment and think about how I was lucky to be alive, that I was still here. I was still breathing. I could fully appreciate being in nature. Swimming in nature strips back and simplifies the material world. It stops my mind wondering. It focuses my breath. It stops me worrying about things that don't matter and allows me to be present in that moment."

Reborn, Laura founded We Swim Wild, a nonprofit organization and public advocacy group dedicated to promoting and protecting wild waters and wild spaces across the United Kingdom. She is currently swimming across all of the UK's national parks to raise awareness about microplastic pollution and other environmental issues.

Nikki Marshall recently wrote eloquently about her fibromyalgia in *The Guardian*. "For me, a flare-up starts with a wave of exhaustion that can swamp me within seconds, accompanied by a brain fog so dense I might struggle to speak. Then the pain begins. It's a rusty feeling in my hands and feet that moves up and seeps into my wrists and ankles, elbows and knees, shoulders and hips. There are muscle aches too, that trampled feeling you get as you're coming down with a cold or flu."

Compounding Nikki's fibromyalgia-related pain is her forty-year-old battle with endometriosis, a debilitating combination she describes as "grinding and relentless and exhausting." So relentless, in fact, she can only recall two days in all of 2021 that were pain-free. "It's never agony . . . but rather whole-body discomfort that steamrollers me. So, I lie down and breathe and wait for sleep to come."

To cope, she takes a daily dose of amitriptyline, an antidepressant that helps block her brain's perception of pain, practices mindful breathing techniques, and gets plenty of rest. She also makes sure she eats a strict anti-inflammatory diet and always walks at least seventy-five hundred steps a day. When she started taking ice baths, she said she hated them at first ("they were horrendous"), but she admits they now leave her feeling "revved up and exhilarated for days."

Like Laura and Nikki, Martin, a sixty-seven-year-old health and safety advisor, discovered that open water can have life-changing effects. "I suffered from health anxiety and depression for most of my life," the grandfather of four told me. "Which means I have spent most of my life focusing on my health, and the fear of being seriously ill and dying. One of the underlying factors was the physical pains throughout my entire body. For years, I was taking antidepression medication, using alcohol and all types of therapies and distractions to mask my pain and fear."

Masking helped, until it didn't. Martin is hardly unique in this. Ultimately, his preferred coping strategy precipitated "a catastrophic mental breakdown," which stemmed from the trauma of watching his sister die when he was younger and a near-death experience of his own. As part of his recovery, he started a strict regimen of walking, which proved promising, until he experienced pains in his fingers and shoulders. After consulting with a rheumatoid arthritis consultant at a local hospital, he was finally diagnosed with fibromyalgia.

In 2016, he says, "I started swimming in a pool. Swimming first thing in the morning gave me some form of exercise and helped with my mental health."

At the same time, however, his fibromyalgia worsened. To help manage his joint pain, his osteopath suggested somatic pilates, which invites practitioners to focus on their inner experience while moving their limbs. In 2020, when his local pilates classes were canceled during the COVID-19 pandemic, he joined the first Chill Therapy group, hoping that it would at least help him manage his mental health. But he got more than he bargained for. Martin says, "After the first session of cold water immersion, I got relief from joint pains for most of the day."

Interestingly, heat, not cold, is usually recommended for reducing the symptoms of fibromyalgia—a hot water bottle, hot baths or showers, or soaking hands or feet in hot water. Typically, this helps reduce pain and alleviate joint stiffness, particularly in the morning. Used to heat treatments, Martin felt nothing but "shock, fear, breathlessness, then a numbness," when he first dipped his foot into the frigid, gray waters of the Atlantic Ocean.

Yet by the time he got out, he felt "alert, alive, and a sense of euphoria and achievement." This shocked him. There was "no pain, no stiffness, only a sense of being one with my body. Suffering from health anxiety and depression all my life, 'being in the moment' was an alien concept. Immersing myself into cold water, however, just puts you there."

A year later, Martin was meeting three times a week with "a bunch of great swimmers and dippers" and finding that "I'm still getting the benefits of cold water." Yet maybe the most profound moment occurred around his third Chill Therapy session, when Martin distinctly recalls floating in the water and feeling, for the first time in decades, a sense of freedom and hope. He says:

> I was looking up at the sky. It was so big and so wide. And the expanse of the sea just filled my mind with calm. The sea brings me back to reality. Its vastness and power remind me just how insignificant my worries are. Not to say that they become irrelevant; more that they become manageable.
>
> The exhilaration, the buzz, the boost to my mood, connection with nature, and the shift of perspective have utterly convinced me that sea swimming has a vital role in looking after my mental health for the future. Feeling a part of something so significant reminds me that any problems I face are relatively small and can be dealt with. This is particularly important for me as a person who catastrophizes about things.
>
> I have never in my wildest dreams thought I could get into the sea in the winter. I thought this would be bad for me, make me ill. But I still cannot believe that I have been going into the sea, two or three times a week since the end of October 2020. Every time I do—even on those dark, wet days—the sense of overwhelming achievement is a priceless drug.

Yet maybe the most profound moment occurred around his third Chill Therapy session, when Martin distinctly recalls floating in the water and feeling, for the first time in decades, a sense of freedom and hope.

CHAPTER 10

"I FEEL HAPPY, I FEEL STRONG, AND I FEEL WHOLE"

Autoimmune Diseases

CROHN'S DISEASE IS A SERIOUS ILLNESS. Any part of the small or large intestine can be involved with varying degrees of severity. An estimated 75 percent of sufferers will, at some time, require surgery directly related to the condition. The wide range of procedures people may have to undergo include the removal of large sections of the bowel and the formation of colostomies and ileostomies. There is also an increased risk of bowel cancer.

Along with ulcerative colitis, Crohn's is one of the two forms of inflammatory bowel disease (IBD) characterized by chronic and prolonged inflammation of the gastrointestinal tract, which can result in permanent damage to the gut. These are distinct from the more common condition known as irritable bowel syndrome

(IBS), which affects the large intestine but has a much better prognosis.

While the exact cause of inflammatory bowel disease is unknown, we do know it is the result of a defective immune system. To protect the body, a properly functioning immune system attacks foreign organisms like viruses and bacteria. Inflammatory bowel disease is the result of the immune system responding incorrectly to environmental triggers, causing it to attack itself. In other words, the defect lies in the immune system's inability to distinguish between itself and invading microorganisms, which is what defines an "autoimmune" disease. There are numerous examples of this, many of which appear to be more and more common, including food allergies, hay fever, and rheumatoid arthritis.

Under ideal conditions, inflammation is a part of a healthy immune system. Like most things in life, though, it's possible to have too much of a good thing. A consequence of the immune system's overactive misfiring, inflammation in the gastrointestinal tract, explains why the condition is also associated with inflammation of skin, eyes, joints, liver, bile ducts, and kidneys, which results in kidney stones.

A recent review and meta-analysis published in *The Lancet* points to a high prevalence of anxiety and depression symptoms in patients with inflammatory bowel disease. In the study, about a third of patients were affected by symptoms of anxiety, and a quarter were affected by symptoms of depression. The prevalence of these symptoms increased in patients with active disease: Half of these patients met the study's criteria for symptoms of anxiety, while a third for symptoms of depression.

IBD and other autoimmune diseases are all-consuming, affecting nearly every aspect of a person's mental and physical well-being.

Over the course of my career, I have anesthetized many patients undergoing operations for IBD. I remember one quite clearly. The patient was a delightful woman in her early twenties. She was scheduled for a laparotomy, an abdominal surgery to remove a length of her bowel, and a colostomy. I was a newly appointed consultant—still in my thirties, just a little older than the patient—and I was struck by how incredibly slim she was. This was, at least partially, due to malnutrition, a consequence of her illness, which reduced her intestine's ability to absorb nutrients. In addition to administering general anesthesia, standard practice for a laparotomy is to insert an epidural catheter, which provides pain relief and attenuates the stress response to surgery.

One of the possible complications, however, is something known as a "dural tap" or spinal puncture. (A spinal tap, as well as being the name of a fictional rock band, is an entirely different procedure.) When this happens, a large quantity of cerebrospinal fluid, which bathes the spinal cord, is released, and patients often end up with a severe headache. As I approached the woman's back, I remember thinking how careful I needed to be to avoid this complication. Generally, the distance to encounter the epidural space is 5 to 6 centimeters; going any further reaches the spinal space. In over a quarter of a century as an anesthetist, the shortest distance I have otherwise encountered is 3.5 to 4 centimeters. In this woman's case, I put the needle in barely 2 centimeters and was greeted with a gush of cerebrospinal fluid. This is a perfect illustration of the effects of IBD on the health of a young woman.

DOMINATING DAILY LIFE

Any kind of IBD is brutal, and it's particularly dreadful for children suffering severe abdominal pain and cramps, frequent diarrhea, blood in their stool, and the consequent fatigue that wipes them out for hours.

It's worse and really confusing for a child if adults don't understand what's going on either. Too often, a child or young adult with IBD can be misdiagnosed with an eating disorder, and they're often put on medication to force them to eat because their weight is so low. This was at least better than the 1930s, when doctors misunderstood the cause and sometimes lobotomized patients in a misguided attempt to cure it. But as recently as the 1970s, when Rob Starr was growing up, Crohn's disease—even when recognized—had no effective treatment.

"My illness stopped me concentrating at school because of the pain," Rob told me. "I was considered lazy and disruptive. But my condition was not a thing back then, so I was just seen as a naughty kid. This, I think, definitely made me perform badly at school, and because I was labeled as such, I lived up to my reputation. I left school just before my sixteenth birthday."

After dropping out, Rob moved forward, refusing to feel sorry for himself or suffer in his solitude at home. He landed an entry-level job at a local insurance company in Brighton, essentially a low-paid internship. "The owner liked me and said I could make tea and coffee."

Over time, Rob worked his way up the proverbial ladder, eventually taking over responsibilities for a poor-performing sales rep. "I had been listening to everyone on the phone and the front desk and had really soaked it all up and made myself employable by him."

However, as his career started to take off, his condition deteriorated.

"It was when I was about twenty my weight suddenly dropped dramatically," Rob says. "I went to visit my parents at their house, and I couldn't make it up the stairs. I was unable to control my bowel movements, which was rather unpleasant for me. I was taken to hospital and put on an IV. I was in intensive care for about twelve weeks because they couldn't diagnose my problem and I was unable to eat." As a result, Rob's weight dropped below eighty-four pounds (six stone).

Eventually, some smart doctor diagnosed Rob with Crohn's.

To cope, he took a complex cocktail of the steroid prednisolone, which helped reduce his inflammation, and the immunosuppressant mercaptopurine, which is also prescribed to treat specific types of blood-related cancers, including leukemia. While the medications stabilized his condition, they came with a brutal series of side effects. His mercaptopurine pills suppressed his bone marrow, which limited his body's natural ability to manufacture blood cells. The drugs also led to liver toxicity and vomiting and loss of appetite, the exact opposite of what someone wants when they're struggling to maintain a healthy weight. In total, Rob was taking four mecaptopurine pills a day on top of almost inconceivable quantities of prednisolone, from six pills a day to more than forty pills a day at his lowest points.

He also developed osteoporosis due to his medication; this was diagnosed when a break in his wrist never fully healed. A scan to check his bone density showed his spine had the density of a ninety-year-old man.

As if these physical ailments weren't bad enough, Rob experienced inflammation in his joints, eyes, and liver. The consequence of the latter was that he was no longer able to excrete uric acid—a toxic metabolite—which then built up in and around his joints. "My arthritis was diagnosed because I had a number of times when I was unable to walk due to very severe pain and swelling. I also had lesions on all my fingers and my feet and needed to have them burnt off by an open flame every three weeks. This meant one week out of every four I had no use of my hands and feet, as they were swollen from the burning. I had dry eyes, which means they had to put little things into my eye ducts to allow the water to flow."

Like so many sufferers of IBD, Rob felt as if his condition dominated his life.

But ever the optimist, Rob continued to move forward. He took up sports, against the advice of his doctors, who told him he could end up breaking his spine. Squash, running, cycling—he did anything that didn't cause too much pain. At the same time, he set up the Starr Trust charity to help disadvantaged kids. This act of altruism inadvertently introduced him to the benefits of ocean swimming.

Initially, Rob wanted to run a marathon and raise money for the charity, but the Crohn's prevented him from running longer distances. "I still wanted to do something," he says. "I was watching TV and saw a story about a channel swimmer. I decided to swim to France instead. I was a nonswimmer pretty much, and I expected my Crohn's to stop me, but I gave it a go. I was still on the Crohn's pills when I began."

"THE BEST THING EVER": ROB'S COLD WATER SWIM CURE

For many illnesses, exercise is a great intervention, in part because it helps reduce inflammation in the body. Potentially, this could help mitigate the bowel symptoms and associated effects of Crohn's. Unfortunately, exercise can be quite difficult or even risky for people with IBD, which is why Rob's doctor recommended against it. It is difficult to absorb the nutrients required to be athletic at any significant level, as the story of the young woman I anesthetized demonstrates. Worse, he risked further and more serious bone fractures. With IBD, some cures can be worse than the condition.

Rob recalls his first few times in the water. As with other first-time, cold water swimmers, the first swim was shocking. The second and third swims weren't as bad. By his seventh swim, Rob recalls, it became "the best thing ever."

"It was about a month or so into my sea swimming that I realized I was going to the beach in pain—mornings are always worst—but that the pain would fade and I would be fine until maybe bedtime or even the next morning. Also, if I was suffering from my arthritis, I would be pain-free all the time I was in the water, which was a massive relief."

Rob started documenting his pain, pre- and postswim. Seeing the effect in black-and-white cemented his resolve to quit his medication—a radical step. "I didn't tell anyone, not even my wife," he says. "I would shake the pill bottles in the bathroom so it sounded like I was taking pills and then I would flush them away—pathetic at my age! After a couple of months, I found I was in pain in the mornings, but once I was in the sea, it was gone until the next day. I took a couple of weeks off swimming to just be certain, and almost instantly, my pain was back throughout the day. Without pills and without swimming, I was struggling throughout the day. My weight was falling off again, and it was just hard to be me. After two weeks I went back to the sea and, hey presto! All was well again."

A solo swim of the English Channel is a massive undertaking. I've done a fair number of open-water swims over five miles, and whenever I do, people suggest that I try my own solo channel swim. My reply is that I swim outdoors for fun. There is nothing fun about spending up to twenty-four hours in the cold, often feeling seasick, and simultaneously worried about the constant threat of jellyfish and container ship traffic. There's not even a good view, and when you get to France, rather than stopping for a celebratory gourmet meal and a glass of champagne, you have to clamber onto the same small fishing boat that guided you from the English coast and head straight back to Dover.

Furthermore, the training is brutal. I get by on a couple of good ninety-minute pool sessions with a really good coach every week, along with a daily cycle to work and dips in the ocean. That total wouldn't even be sufficient for a single channel training session. Then, to even qualify to do an official channel crossing you have to complete a six-hour qualifying swim in water that is 60°F (15°C) or less. It takes hours and hours in both the pool and open water, sucking down energy drinks and fueling on gummies and flapjacks. (Actually, that last one is pretty good—Rob and I have a mutual friend, Fiona, who has coached many successful crossings and makes the best flapjacks in the world.)

As Rob upped his training to these inhuman levels, his Crohn's deteriorated, and unable to refuel properly (despite access to Fiona's baking skills), his weight plummeted again, which forced him to cut back on his training. Once again, we see that too much of a good thing can turn bad.

Rob trained solidly for two years but could never get beyond an eight-hour swim, so he adapted and joined a relay-team channel crossing. The team managed to make it to France in August 2012, in the process raising over £80,000 (or about $106,000), which funded twenty-one projects helping young people.

Rob says, "I also found that it was amazing for my head! I was under a lot of stress when I took this up. I was dealing with my illnesses, I had a six-month-old baby, I was building our family house, I was running a business and a charity, and I had just lost my dad at age sixty from cancer. And of course, I was starting training for an event that would challenge me physically and mentally in every way. But somehow, when I was in the sea, all my worries and stresses floated away. I am not sure I could have coped with everything at that time if I did not have the calmness of the sea every morning."

His arthritis, which previously used to cause bouts of painful swelling almost every week, now only affects him around six times a year. And the painful lesions on his hands and feet—and the necessity to burn them off—went away once he stopped taking his medications and took up cold water swimming.

These days, when Rob is unable to access open water, his symptoms return: After a few days, he develops abdominal pains, and if he goes more than a week without swimming, his pain feels similar to his previous flare-ups.

While Rob isn't one to overindulge, he is often tempted to have a treat that he knows will challenge his constitution. He knows he can get away with it, though, because any discomfort will be gone by the time he's walking back up the beach following his daily "constitutional."

I am not sure I could have coped
with everything at that time if
I did not have the calmness of
the sea every morning.

Today, Rob only takes one pill a day for his arthritis. He still suffers from almost daily diarrhea and pain, which can wipe him out for a couple of hours, but he has found the resolve to compete and take on almost Herculean challenges. "I have managed to run full marathons, cycle up Le Mont Ventoux, complete a dozen Olympic triathlons, and two half-Ironman competitions." Then, in the summer of 2021, he successfully completed a full Ironman in just under fourteen hours. When I think of the twenty-year-old kid who was unable to walk up his parents' stairs, I find this utterly incredible. After his full Ironman, he told me he was back in the ocean the following morning, enjoying the water lapping over his aching body.

Rob says that he went "quite deep into mindfulness and taught myself meditation and how to close my mind off from the world and from pain in general. It might sound a bit crazy, but I actually can turn off pain by just breathing and zeroing it out. However, I would absolutely not have been able to do these things if I did not have the sea to keep my illnesses under control."

The effects are not simply physical. Rob says:

> Over the years I have used the sea as my form of meditation. Every worry or stress that I have is dealt with in my mind by swimming them away. The sea has not only become my physical medication but also my mental savior. I cannot stress enough how important my sea swimming is to me.

I feel happy, I feel strong, and I feel whole. The feeling of freedom and being out in nature first thing in the morning is just an incredible way to start the day. I can only guess what it is about the cold water that makes a difference! It certainly takes my mind off other things—such as physical pain or mental pain. Maybe it's the cold, or the movement of the sea, or the natural chemicals, or all the above. But whatever it is, it is incredible.

Sea swimming literally has transformed every aspect of who I am.

CHAPTER 11

"IT HELPS ME FEEL GROUNDED AND STRONG"

Trauma and Post-Traumatic Stress Disorder

"LIFE," BUDDHA TELLS US, "IS SUFFERING."

Stress is inevitable. We all have to deal with it, usually on a daily basis. Most of the time it ebbs and flows. But because the lower limit of the ebb can be too high, stress has a chronic, deleterious effect on our health. Once again, the principal mechanism through which this is mediated is inflammation.

Ongoing mental stress chronically raises blood levels of stress hormones, in particular, cortisol. Cortisol is referred to as nature's built-in alarm system, and its secretion is an essential part of our defense mechanism. It has a wide range of effects, which includes raising blood sugar levels, priming our white blood cells for action, and releasing pro-inflammatory molecules in order to prepare the body for physical injury or infection. However, while these effects are positive in an acute situation, with long-term stress, levels can remain high in the absence of a physical threat and this results in damage to our tissues.

We all suffer emotional and physical trauma in our lives, whether it's losing our job, someone close to us dying, or failing at school. There is a spectrum of trauma and a spectrum of reactions.

The American Psychological Association describes trauma as an emotional response to a terrible event. Shock and denial are typical in the immediate aftermath. Later, reactions include unpredictable emotions, flashbacks, strained relationships, and physical symptoms like headaches and nausea.

All of these feelings and reactions to traumatic events are expected.

"Adjustment disorder" occurs when the emotional or behavioral symptoms a person experiences are more severe than would be expected. While the symptoms themselves might seem appropriate—such as feeling tense, sad, or hopeless; withdrawing from other people; acting defiantly or showing impulsive behavior; and physical manifestations like tremors, palpitations, and headaches—in combination they can become overwhelming and cause significant distress.

This is very common. Around 5 to 20 percent of individuals receiving outpatient mental health treatment have a principal diagnosis of adjustment disorder, and more than 15 percent of adults with cancer develop adjustment disorder.

When a breakdown occurs in relation to a single traumatic event, it's termed "acute stress disorder." Typically, the symptoms occur between three days and one month after the event and include flashbacks, nightmares, and feeling numb and detached. An estimated 21 percent of survivors of car accidents develop acute stress disorder, and between 20 and 50 percent of survivors of assault, rape, or mass shootings develop it.

When the symptoms last for more than a month and cause significant distress or problems in someone's daily functioning, it is classified as post-traumatic stress disorder (PTSD), a state of heightened arousal and disproportionate reactivity. About half of people with acute stress disorder develop PTSD, which affects approximately 3.5 percent of US and UK adults every year. Shockingly, an estimated one in eleven people will be diagnosed with PTSD in their lifetime—and women are twice as likely as men to have PTSD.

People with PTSD describe flashbacks so vivid they feel as if the traumatic event is occurring again in the present. Furthermore, they describe experiencing a hyperawareness of sounds, smells, or tastes connected to the trauma, along with physical sensations of pain, pressure, sweating, or nausea that can last from a few seconds to hours or even days. Here's how one person vividly described the experience: "My heart was constantly racing, and I felt permanently dizzy. I couldn't leave the house and became afraid of going to sleep, as I was convinced I was going to die."

When someone is reminded of the traumatic event, reactions include panicking, getting upset or angry easily, hypervigilance, and poor or insufficient sleep, which results in irritability or aggressive behavior. As another sufferer said, "The lack of sleep and the sense of never being at peace are exhausting."

To make things worse, people with PTSD can often have difficulty expressing affection, and they can exhibit self-destructive or reckless behavior, like abusing drugs and alcohol. Another person reflected: "My behavior changed and became erratic. I would alternate from wanting to shut myself away and not see or talk to anyone to going out to parties in the middle of the week and staying out late." Another sufferer shared how trauma can emerge weeks or months after the triggering event: "I thought I was coping quite well to start with. Then a few weeks after the event, I began experiencing unpleasant physical symptoms, similar to those of a heart attack: chest pain, tightness, and dizzy spells so severe that I thought I would pass out."

The origin of these reoccurring physical effects relates to the body's response to stress. The body releases cortisol and adrenaline to respond to a threat. When a person remembers a previous traumatic experience, since the memory is so strong, it again triggers the same stress reaction: fight, flight, or freeze. Fight and flight are forms of mobilization, when we respond by defending ourselves or escaping to survive a danger. Freeze or immobilization is a kind of paralysis, when we experience too much stress to do anything. When the nervous system is unable to return to its normal state of balance, this prevents someone from moving past—or moving on from—the initial traumatic event. The working theory is that people who suffer the ongoing psychological effects of stress and trauma, whether they develop PTSD or not, store experiences in ways that are not processed appropriately. While many will recover quickly, a significant number won't. Those who do not recover require some kind of resetting of their neurological circuits.

At present, active therapies for trauma and PTSD include cognitive behavioral therapy and EMDR, or eye movement desensitization and reprocessing. Many sufferers also have coexisting mental health issues, including depression, which can require medication. Nevertheless, while medications can help, they may also exacerbate feeling emotionally numb and cut off.

There is a lot we can do on our own to help ourselves cope with stress and the ongoing impact of traumatic events. These include the following five simple, self-directed interventions:

1. Get moving and exercise, particularly by walking, running, cycling, and swimming.
2. Participate in social activities in order to feel part of a community.
3. Practice mindfulness and deep, controlled breathing to regulate emotions.
4. Take good care to eat and sleep well.
5. Connect with nature and the outdoors.

Of course, all these things can be achieved by joining an open water swimming group.

MENTAL HEALTH SWIMS: RACHEL'S COLD WATER SWIM CURE

One person who can attest to this approach is Rachel Ashe, a wonderful, resilient young woman who has dealt with several mental health issues since childhood.

"I was adopted as a baby," Rachel told me. "I'm not sure if this made me more vulnerable than others, but I was really unlucky. I experienced grooming, sexual abuse, and rape from multiple people during my childhood and, later, as a young adult. I tried to kill myself when I was fourteen, then got very involved in drugs because I wanted to feel something that wasn't deeply sad. My family are middle-class stiff-upper-lippers who didn't used to talk about feelings, so I didn't really know how to tell anyone how bad things were."

Rachel describes the consequences of this trauma: "My self-confidence was badly knocked, my ability to know who is safe and who isn't, which resulted in trust issues, disassociation, nightmares, insomnia, struggles with school, and then later, at university and work."

Among her litany of mental health issues are post-traumatic stress disorder, avoidant personality disorder, emotionally unstable personality disorder, social anxiety, and depression. To deal with them, she turned to therapy, running, and medication prescribed by her psychiatrist, including antipsychotics, zopiclone, diazepam, and antidepressants. She also explored meditation, breathing exercises, and other mindfulness practices, but these only worsened her symptoms of disassociation. And she tried self-medicating with illicit drugs.

Nothing, however, really worked until she started cold water swimming.

Adapting to the shock of the cold would give her body and mind some purchase over her parasympathetic nervous system, which would slow down her heart rate and diminish her stress response, both to past and present events alike. Open water swimming has the ability to shift our consciousness away from the incessant, frequently negative mental chatter and ground us in the physical present moment.

Swimming also helped Rachel reconnect to more enjoyable experiences from her youth in Portobello, a small seaside suburb in Edinburgh, where her passion for watery places began. "I fell asleep to the sound of the waves every night and played on the beach in all weathers as a child. When I was wee, I remember dancing through puddles on the prom during an autumn storm. It was raining so much it was really dark. I was soaked to the skin but felt the happiest I had ever felt before. As a child, having picnics, going for walks, and swimming in the rain, surrounded by midges, was not unusual. I was one of those kids who always got wet no matter what we were doing. I loved water and mud with a passion."

Many years later, she spontaneously decided to join the annual New Year's dip on the Portobello beach she remembered so well from her childhood.

Nothing, however, really worked until she started cold water swimming.

"It was really bloody cold," she recalls. "It felt like my skin was burning, and I wanted to get out straight away."

Despite only staying in the water for less than a minute, she felt an incredible calm come over her as she exited the water. After this first swim, she was hooked. She continued her cold water swimming every month that year. Swimming complemented her ongoing intensive therapy sessions.

"It helps me connect with myself, with others, and with nature," Rachel says. "It helps me feel grounded and strong. When I'm feeling anxious or zoned out, cold water works almost instantly. On bad days, I really don't want to get out of the water because it makes such a difference to how I feel. It forces me to be present in my body. There is nothing else but the cold. It usually kicks in as I'm walking back up the beach. I feel the soles of my feet on the sand. I feel the wind. And instead of feeling like my mind is wandering, I feel like mind and body are united and capable again."

After two years of this "life-changing" therapy, she now feels empowered, a more developed, healthier, and healed adult in the prime of her life. "I can now say I am creative, imaginative, driven, and passionate. I used to wear a smiley mask all the time and didn't want anyone to know how screwed up I felt on the inside. It was exhausting."

Not only has Rachel benefited from cold water swimming, she has introduced the practice and its benefits to hundreds of others by setting up Mental Health Swims, a community that "welcomes and empowers everyone—people of all body shapes, skin colors, ages, backgrounds, genders, sexualities, and abilities—to enjoy the healing power of cold water and community."

This organization started with a simple post she put out on social media in September 2019, which resulted in nearly thirty people joining her for a swim. "It's an easygoing group," according to Rachel, "that favors short dips to long distances and prides companionship over competition. Participants can either chat on the beach or swim in the shallows, whatever works best for them."

For Rachel, swimming "meant I was getting out of the house early in the morning to have a dip before work; it opened the world up for me. I wanted to share that pleasure with as many people as possible.

"But I think rather than swimming changing my life, it was setting up a community that welcomed everyone, no matter how they're feeling, which really made the difference. I wanted to create a safe space for people to come as they feel without judgment or shame."

"A SEA OF SILENT EUPHORIA": SWITCHING FROM LEFT BRAIN TO RIGHT BRAIN

The cause of the profoundly transformative effect of cold water swimming on the mind is, for now, beyond the reach of neuroscience. The deepest insight and the nearest I've come to an explanation derives from the extraordinary experiences and work of American neuroscientist Jill Bolte Taylor. While working in a

Harvard Medical School neuroscience lab, she experienced what she describes as "nirvana," a breakthrough about how the brain works. She experienced this nirvana by having a stroke—an event she has chronicled in a TED Talk, which has been viewed more than twenty-five million times, and in her bestselling book *My Stroke of Insight*.

Based on her research and experience, Bolte Taylor proposes that the brain creates our "selves" by combining four distinct characters, which can be delineated anatomically—two from the left brain and two from the right. The left side of our brain, Bolte Taylor explains, thinks linearly, logically, and methodically. It gives us our sense of time and, as a result, our sense of the past and the future. She has said the left side of our brain is "designed to take that enormous collage of the present moment and start picking out details, and more details about those details." Then the left side "categorizes and organizes all that information, associates it with everything in the past we've ever learned, and projects into the future all of our possibilities." Because the left side of our brain thinks in language, according to Bolte Taylor, it connects us and our internal world to our external world.

The left brain is subdivided into two distinct parts: one rational and one fear-based. One part establishes the boundary of our body and creates the sense of self that allows us to interact and communicate with the external world. The second part integrates all those details, projects into the future, and protects us by generating fear.

Conversely, our right hemisphere thinks in pictures and learns kinesthetically, or through the movement of our bodies. "Information, in the form of energy, streams in simultaneously through all of our sensory systems," Bolte Taylor summarizes in her wildly popular TED Talk, "and then it explodes into this enormous collage of what this present moment looks like, what this present moment smells like and tastes like, what it feels like and what it sounds like. I am an energy-being connected to the energy all around me through the consciousness of my right hemisphere. We are energy-beings connected to one another through the consciousness of our right hemispheres as one human family."

Creativity and empathy come from the right side of the brain, which is also subdivided into two parts: one focused on the moment and one empathetic. One part lets us have fun with no thought of the consequences, which is the sole concern of the left brain. The second part gives us a boundaryless connection of empathy with the universe.

The blood vessel that burst in Bolte Taylor's brain was located on the left side. The incident produced a clot the size of a golf ball. "As soon as my left hemisphere says to me 'I am,' I become separate. I become a single solid individual, separate from the energy flow around me and separate from you. And this was the portion of my brain that I lost on the morning of my stroke."

Immediately, ego, analysis, judgment, and context began to fail her.

Oddly, although she realized in the moment that she was experiencing a critical medical emergency, she says it felt great. The incessant chatter and everyday concerns that normally filled her mind disappeared. Her perception changed to such a degree she felt that the atoms and molecules making up her body blended with the space around her. The whole world, and all the creatures in it, were part of the same magnificent field of shimmering energy.

"My perception of physical boundaries was no longer limited to where my skin met air. . . . I felt like a genie liberated from its bottle. The energy of my spirit seemed to flow like a great whale gliding through a sea of silent euphoria."

It took an almost insurmountable struggle to get help, and afterward, Bolte Taylor required surgery and eight years of rehabilitation to get back to being able to live a normal life again. Throughout, she was driven by the desire to communicate the insights she had gained to help people live a more peaceful life with a more "balanced brain," as she calls it. To accomplish this, she started promoting techniques that "take a step to the right."

Watching her TED Talk, and hearing her on Mo Gawdat's wonderful *Slo Mo* podcast, I was struck by the parallels with my own experience of the effect of cold water: the disappearance of mental chatter and worries. The switch from the past and future to the immediate present. The energy of my spirit. The euphoria. Although, physically, I am more like a beached whale, spiritually I am definitely "gliding through a sea of silent euphoria."

By taking us completely into the moment and producing that feeling of connection with the people around us and our environment, cold water swimming breaks those endless loops and subdues the fears our left brain is constantly feeding us.

"CALMER, GENTLER, WHOLE AGAIN": SAM'S COLD WATER SWIM CURE

Like Rachel, Sam Murray found peace in cold water.

A former Royal Marine in the British Army, he was diagnosed with PTSD after serving nine years in the military. "To make the pain go away," he told me, "I drank and drank and drank. I was in a really dark place."

After several failed suicide attempts, he was checked into a psychiatric facility, where he was pumped so full of medications, he barely recalls his first month there. Talk therapy sessions helped him start to address the past traumas that triggered his PTSD, but he ultimately felt as if he was only scratching old wounds, rather than moving past them. Antidepressants also weren't working for him. That's when he realized he needed to do something radical and immediate, something that made more sense for him. To find it, he set out on a journey of reflection, contemplation, and self-discovery.

At one point, he took a neurolinguistic programming and hypnotherapy course, which "wasn't really resonating with me," he says, but he was intrigued by a man who practiced a form of breath work every morning before getting in a swimming pool filled with ice. "I decided to give it a try. I was skeptical, but I did three rounds of breath work and swimming. Straight away, I experienced an awakening. I woke up. Not in a religious sense, just in a new awareness of life, in the here and now."

That was September 2019.

According to Sam, he's gone in the water every day since. "I know the massive impact. I don't use antidepressants and I don't use alcohol anymore. Or anything else. I just use the cold water. It keeps me alive."

People are constantly amazed at his transformation. They note he's hardly the same Sam who used to drink two bottles of wine and do whatever drugs he could get his hands on. He's a better version of himself—calmer, gentler, whole again.

"The reason I love cold water swimming is because it instantly brings me into the present. My mind clears of any worries of the past or a future that doesn't even exist. I become at one with everything around me. I have the most amazing feeling of connection, with nature and my own self."

Sam's experiences parallel Jill Bolte Taylor's left brain/right brain switch, as well as the reorientating sensation I and countless other cold water swimmers experience in and out of the water. Cold water interrupts the tendency to dwell on our most harrowing and most intimate thoughts, which empowers us to break reoccurring cycles of overthinking, anxiety, trauma, and PTSD. When we emerge from the challenge of swimming in cold water, we inevitably find that our emotional state has shifted from fearful and angsty toward excited and happy.

In addition to finding peace in the water, Sam also found his purpose.

Along with his partner, a nutritional therapist and breath-work practitioner, he developed a form of therapy that combines diaphragmatic breathing, meditation, and cold water swimming. This technique serves as the foundation of their organization Breath Connection (see "Websites and Organizations," page 224), which they started primarily to help veterans like Sam and frontline personnel cope with stress and anxiety and overcome their traumas.

Sam explains:

> We get them into their bodies and out of their heads. I feel that breath work and cold water is particularly ideal for veterans and serving members of the armed forces because both practices have a big impact on the nervous system. If you practice the techniques regularly, it improves vagal tone (stimulating the vagus nerve and the parasympathetic nervous system) and helps build resilience. Breath work and cold water swimming also lower inflammation and support greater blood flow and oxygen transport, which is ideal for healing old injuries.
>
> It's all about the immersion and getting out and getting all the benefits that they need. Then they've got a sense of achievement. They feel, you know, really proud that they've done it. They feel as if they've won the day.

CHAPTER 12

"SWIMMING AND SOCIALIZING HAVE HELPED ME MORE THAN PILLS EVER DID"

Depression and Mental Health

TOWARD THE END OF 2020, I began working for part of the year as an anaesthetist in Kristiansand, Norway. Despite the bitter cold, outdoor swimming is on the increase here as well. During the spring of 2021, I enjoyed a fantastic morning with my friend Solveig (pronounced "sool-vay," which rhymes with "pool play") on Flekkerøy, the island where I live with my family. Together, she and I walked fifteen or twenty minutes through the woods to emerge at a gorgeous, sun-brightened turquoise sea. Its smooth surface was interrupted only by the Oksøy Lighthouse and the rocky outcroppings of ancient metamorphic gneiss with its characteristic banded layers. Beyond these, an endless horizon—Sweden to the east and Denmark to the south.

Enjoying warm drinks from our thermos flasks, we shared stories of our cold water experiences, laughing. When we got in, the water was a balmy 44°F (6.7°C). Well, balmy in comparison to a month earlier, when the temperature was only 33°F (0.3°C) and ice floated on the ocean. We still felt the cold burning our skin and then, best of all, that familiar postswim euphoria. We enjoyed two swims, in fact, because on this occasion we were being filmed for an upcoming Norwegian television show, and the producers wanted to capture our adventure, first with an airborne drone, then with an underwater one.

It has not always been possible for Solveig to enjoy such simple pleasures. For the past thirty years, she has suffered from bipolar disorder.

As a sixteen-year-old, she was outgoing and happy. But then she found herself struggling with sleep and not wanting to hang out with friends so much. This was the start of her first depressive episode. It lasted three months. "From being happy and finding life easy," she says, "I began to wonder how it was possible to even exist."

Struggling with depression throughout her teenage years, Solveig still remained active, exploring her many passions. One was acting. However, when she was twenty-four, she was performing in a play one night and began to overact. As the scenes unfolded, she brazenly hijacked the starring role from the lead actress and started screaming and singing over the lines of other performers. Or at least that was what she was later told. To this day, she has no recollection of it. Following this psychotic episode, she was diagnosed with bipolar disorder, also known as manic depression.

"I had many episodes of psychosis in my twenties, and over the next decade, I was in and out of the psychiatric ward many times," she told me.

Solveig suffered massive swings in her psychological state; during the worst ones, she felt completely removed from her body. Her mind seemed to look at herself from the outside. Once, she was convinced that she was in a film, charged with the power to fly. On another occasion, she believed she was a UFO. On another, she stripped out of her clothes and ran naked around a local park. "It seems surrealistic because it seems so far removed from how I am now. But I know that I often felt like the master of the world, and the things that I did many times during my psychotic episodes are incredibly embarrassing to think of now."

On the other end of these manic episodes were deeply depressive ones, which made her suicidal. "I would read the obituaries and wish that it was my name that was there. I also wished that I was my grandmother because she was old and didn't have so long to live. It was a terrible period. I didn't live, I just existed."

It finally came to the point where she carefully weighed all the options and decided that the only solution was to take an overdose. In 2001, on temporary release from the psychiatric hospital, she put a bucket of water by the side of her bed and took, in her words, a "mountain" of pills. "I had this idea that

I would lose consciousness due to the pills, fall into the bucket, and drown."

Earlier that day, she had visited her mother, who had become worried for her and, fortunately, went to check up on her. When Solveig didn't answer, her mother broke down the door and rushed her to the hospital, where she subsequently underwent a course of electroconvulsive therapy, or ECT. This is a process whereby people suffering from severe depression have an electrical current passed across their brains.

Today, she describes these events as a turning point.

"After I received a course of ECT, I was no longer suicidal, but it's taken many years since then to learn to live with the condition. I still have manic periods, but I handle them better, and today, I am thankful and happy in the life that I have."

Her life now centers on her husband and two children, and she has developed a way of living that keeps her condition under control. "I have to plan each day. It is as if it is a productive job, even though I am on benefits. I am dependent on predictability, and it's important that the calendar isn't too full. It is a balancing act to be able to live well with this condition."

One of the key parts to her regime is spending time outdoors in nature with friends.

Then, a couple of winters ago, one of her friends suggested they go for a swim in a lake in the woods near her house. Her friend had taken up cold water swimming following her husband's terminal cancer diagnosis. Solveig was skeptical. But over time, swimming became a valuable and effective part of her routine, and Norwegian national television, NRK (equivalent to the BBC), was keen to tell her story. Solveig was just as keen to share her experiences as Sarah was to share her experiences with depression. That was why Solveig and I were being filmed that day, and our cold water swim together brought me back to where I started.

UNDERSTANDING DEPRESSION AND THE COLD WATER SWIM CURE

Back in 2004, my experience of how great I felt after a gentle lap around Brighton's Palace Pier set off my curiosity and, ultimately, started me on a quest to uncover the potential health benefits of cold water swimming and explore more deeply the link between depression and inflammation.

Since that moment, I have learned a lot about both the body and the mind and how they are affected by cold water physiology. I have had my eyes opened to the enormous diversity of depression and related mental health issues (anxiety, most especially), their myriad societal causes and effects, the interaction of mental health and physical illness, the difficulty of treating them, and the way the pharmaceutical industry has dictated treatment protocols.

When we can easily delineate the cause and effect of a condition, it can be straightforward to treat. An underactive thyroid gland, for example, produces less of the hormone thyroxine. This can be replaced with a tablet of thyroxine. But most conditions do not have such a discreet cause and simple treatment. The more complex the cause, the more difficult something is to treat, and the brain is inconceivably complex.

Overall, depression tends to be associated with certain changes in the way the brain and body function, but individual cases of depression are distinct. There's no single cause that applies to all cases. Hypothyroidism describes the cause of an illness—low levels of thyroxine—but depression is defined by a cluster of symptoms that, without further context, provide few clues to the cause.

As I discuss in chapter 4, the nearest we can get to a common causative feature of depression is inflammation. People who suffer from depression are about 50 percent more likely to have raised levels of inflammation compared with people who do not suffer from depression, as measured by the blood biomarker C-reactive protein (CRP). However, this still means that about 50 percent of people with depression do not have raised CRP levels.

Despite these caveats, my colleagues and I still felt it was a hypothesis worth exploring.

One morning in September 2020, prior to the start of a two-month Chill Therapy session, we assembled twenty-seven participants on the beach. All were there because they suffered from depression and/or anxiety. Using a new machine that only requires a drop of blood, we measured the CRP levels of each participant before they plunged into the water for the first time. Out of twenty-seven participants, twelve had raised CRP levels. Then, at the end of eight weeks and eight cold water swims, we tested everyone's CRP levels again. Of the twelve participants with elevated levels, nine of them had dropped, two had maintained the same levels, and only one went up. Among the other fifteen swimmers, only one person's CRP levels rose, and even then, the increase was just barely detectable. This result is counterintuitive. The common belief is that stress always raises levels of inflammation, and cold water swimming is definitely stressful, mentally and physically. So this small study suggests that cold immersion—carried out in a sensibly controlled fashion—is, at the very least, unlikely to have a negative impact on inflammation, and it perhaps has a positive effect.

At the same time, it indicates that even the closest we can get to a common causative denominator isn't really that common. This little experiment lends support to the hypothesis that it's unlikely a single treatment modality is going to work for everyone. That said, it is worth noting that there may still be value in measuring CRP levels. This is because there is some evidence inflammatory- and noninflammatory-associated depression respond differently to different treatments. For example, a study of the administration of omega-3 oils on people suffering from depression found that, while the oil didn't seem to have an effect overall, if the depressed patients had elevated levels of inflammation, the treatment worked better than a placebo.

At present, the most prevalent framework for understanding the cause and treatment of mental health disorders remains a biochemical imbalance or deficiency in the brain. As a result, both medical and nonmedical treatments like exercise are directed toward increasing the levels of serotonin, dopamine, noradrenaline, or whatever other neurotransmitters seem to be involved. There is no doubt that neurotransmitters play significant roles in determining our mental state, but given the complexity of the nervous system's circuitry, their contribution is just one part of the whole. It's like describing the world's transport system only in terms of the type of fuel used to power vehicles.

In the brain, there are as many cells as there are observable stars in the Milky Way, about 86 billion. All these cells communicate, which means our brains have an incomprehensible number of 10^{15}—a quadrillion or a million billion—connections. That's not all. Depending on which of the hundred different neurotransmitters is secreted, signals can be further modified. Compare this to the world's most powerful supercomputers, which complete approximately two hundred petaFLOPS (10^{15}) calculations per second. Although it's impossible to calculate accurately, it's estimated that human brains work at the next order higher—at one exaFLOPS (10^{18}) or a billion billion calculations every single second.

Because the brain can perceive, interpret, store, analyze, and redistribute simultaneously, it can process information in a few hundred neural transmissions, whereas a computer with distinct parts for processing and memory requires a few million transmissions between its component parts. As if this incredible raw power isn't enough, the brain is able to constantly rewire itself, an ability known as neuroplasticity. This rewiring is both an advantage and a disadvantage in terms of mental health. It's a disadvantage because dysfunctional circuits can develop and, like ants leaving trails to a source of food, can become reinforced with use. It's an advantage because these circuits can also be reformed, or rerouted, into more helpful circuits.

Really, it's a miracle that the brain doesn't break down more often.

Despite this complicated configuration, we continue to chalk up mental health disorders to an imbalance, or deficiency, in the brain, largely because it's easier to consider a handful of molecules than the billions of neurons and the trillions of constantly changing connections they share.

Ultimately, incomprehensibly complex patterns of electrical activity in the brain affect our mental state, and neurotransmitters like serotonin are merely passive vectors. And as incomprehensible as it is, we could benefit from considering the ways in which we can influence these circuits.

It makes sense that nonpharmacological therapies can modify the brain's electrical circuits, since these therapies work on a global rather than a molecular level. While these methods can be very nonspecific—such as going for a walk, spending time with friends, or singing in a choir—activities can also be more specifically directed toward improving mental health, whether it's art therapy or cognitive behavioral therapy.

A condition like depression with multiple potential causes is bound to produce multiple targets for treatment. When we don't know the exact physical or psychological cause—if we can even make this distinction—we are in a bit of a therapeutic quandary. It's unlikely that focusing on a single target is going to be especially effective. Another option would be to approach many individual targets with many individual treatments. However, because we are unable to measure levels of neurotransmitters in the brain, it is impossible to know which treatments to use. Another option is to find a single treatment that works on multiple targets—preferably an intervention that works simultaneously on both mind and body.

Cold water could just be that.

Part of Solveig's problem was, in her twenties, she didn't always take her medication. Nowadays, she understands that she is always likely to need some form of medication. Since she began outdoor swimming, however, she has been able to reduce the number of pills she has to take. And after a swim, she feels calmer and happier and sleeps better.

ATARAXIA: CALM AND EQUANIMITY

While cold water swimming isn't going to be a complete cure or even an appropriate treatment for all people with depression and anxiety, by virtue of its multifaceted effects, it is certainly worth considering. Furthermore, with its other physical benefits, it is something to consider before taking pharmaceuticals. Cold water swimming may help curtail the progression from physiological low mood to pathological depression.

Cold water swimming may help curtail the progression from physiological low mood to pathological depression.

Cold water swimming certainly has the potential, over both the short- and long-term, to help boost mental health and catalyze the feelings of reorientation, transformation, and connection that Sarah, Kirsti, Solveig, and many others have described—a result that continues to be borne out by subsequent outdoor swimming surveys and feedback from the Chill Therapy courses.

For instance, the 2019 survey we conducted online through the Outdoor Swimming Society showed that, after a swim outdoors, many people felt an immediate improvement in their mental health, an effect that persisted for up to a week. These results have been published in the *Journal of Medical Internet Research*, and they showed that the probability of outdoor swimming having "some impact" on mental health conditions, including anxiety and PTSD, was forty-four times higher compared to no impact.

Of the 287 swimmers who said they suffered from depression, nearly three-quarters (68.6 percent, or 197 people) said they had been living with their depression for at least ten years. In total, 255 people reported that swimming had a positive impact on their depression, an incredible 88.9 percent. In contrast, only 24 people, or 8.4 percent, said there were no changes to their condition. Interestingly, 87.5 percent of respondents (251 people) said they experienced a continued reduction in symptoms if they swam regularly. The effect of a swim lasted for "hours" in nearly half of the swimmers, but a quarter experienced an effect that lasted one to two days, and there was even a significant proportion, 9.7 percent, in whom the effect lasted for a week or more. Similar levels of effectiveness were also seen in people who were swimming in order to alleviate symptoms of anxiety and post-traumatic stress disorder.

Similarly, a study of Finnish winter swimmers showed a positive outcome in the swimmers' "vigor activity scores," while a study we carried out in swimmers who had joined the Pool2Pier course in Brighton reported increases in vigor and self-esteem, and reductions in negative subscales, including tension, anger, depression, confusion, and total mood disturbance.

More recently, I supervised a morning of cold water–related activities for a group of thirty sixteen- and seventeen-year-old Norwegian schoolchildren, which concluded with a swim in a local lake. Even though it was the students' first time, their scores on the Profile of Mood States questionnaire showed a clear, positive effect.

While I am fairly certain that the anti-inflammatory effect of outdoor swimming is crucial to its beneficial effects on our health, I don't think this alone can explain the way our bodies and minds are transformed by a few minutes in cold water. No doubt some of the euphoria is down to the release of "happy hormones," like adrenaline, noradrenaline, dopamine, oxytocin, and serotonin.

But for me, the most striking and fundamental change between before and after isn't just the high. In Norway, I commute to the hospital where I work by cycling ten miles. Every morning, I enjoy a quick detour to a stunning lake that's right along my route. When

I arrive, my head is always full of chatter, and my body feels tense and heavy. But it never fails: Postswim, as I dry off, I always notice a welcome feeling of clarity, stillness, and looseness. Then, when I'm cruising down the hill for the last leg of my journey, I feel a lightness, possibly even weightlessness. It feels like I'm almost floating above my bike.

In her book *Blue Spaces*, Catherine Kelly relates the words of someone who experiences the water in a similar fashion: "I feel like a tiny little drop floating in the vastness. My tininess doesn't equate to nothingness. On the contrary, it makes me feel like an equal and vital part of one big whole."

When I've asked people what they get from swimming outdoors, they echo these sentiments: "It's like getting rid of the cobwebs"; "the postswim calm is the best feeling." Time and time again, people use words like *connected*, *peace*, and *clarity*. Someone once told me, "Swimming outdoors takes you to another place entirely and frees your mind."

It does. It absolutely takes you to another place, though not as far away as it sometimes seems. It only takes you to the other side of your brain, which is far enough, it seems. Thanks to Jill Bolte Taylor, we know that intense physical sensations take us out of the left brain and into the right so that, as one swimmer recounts, "when the water temperature is in single figures, all I can think about is the cold, exhilaration, and staying afloat. There's no room for all the petty worries about work and chores."

Philosophy has got a reputation for being abstract and too complex for most folks, who don't have time for intellectualism. Drop Nietzsche into the conversation and you've lost your audience. However, some of his greatest insights were the result of his direct observation of the gray-brown mountain cattle that he fell in love with while living in the Swiss Alps. The cattle had a suboptimal existence; life for them was often unpleasant. But in heavy rain and intense sunshine, when flies landed on their noses and their heavy bells chafed their necks, they showed no impatience or anger. They didn't appear to suffer from envy or to regret missed opportunities. They seemed to harbor no plans for revenge or to cower fearfully from the future. He felt they had reached the state of calm and equanimity known to the Greeks as "ataraxia."

Although, intellectually—with my left brain—I'm still not sure what exactly ataraxia means, with my right brain I understand instinctively what it feels like. When I get out of the water, I can totally relate to a patient, calm cow chewing the cud. I experience a brief, welcome, and therapeutic respite before I reenter the reality of hospital work. Ultimately, cold water swimming may not be a "cure" or a complete substitute for medication, but it can complement conventional treatments and work as an effective therapeutic for improved mental health and general well-being—a regular shower of wellness that can bring about radical changes in mind, body, and identity.

CONCLUSION

Be Water

IN 2020 AND 2021, the Outdoor Swimming Society was not able to run its wonderful mass-participation swims due to COVID-related restrictions.

Instead, in 2021, it organized a mass-participation socially and geographically distanced virtual event on June 21, the summer solstice, which was appropriately called "The Longest Swim on the Longest Day."

Seven hundred adults and children from twenty-one different countries around the world participated. The tagline read: "Any stroke, any place, any distance, any age."

I told my son Ib about the upcoming event. He and I were on the beach preparing for one of our winter dips. He looked up and pointed at a small island about two hundred yards away. "Can we swim round that?" he asked.

Perfect, I replied.

It would be his longest open-water swim and our longest swim together.

Midsummer arrived and, with it, came clouds and showers. But that's not the point. Observed by my eldest son, Erik, and barked at by our miniature schnauzer, Lego, we waded in and cast ourselves off.

It was calm. Assisted by his fins, Ib made smooth and swift progress across the water. We chatted as we went. We enjoyed the beauty surrounding us—the coolness of the water, the sound of our steady stroke, the sight of the birds flying overheard, and the sheer pleasure of physical activity. Our swim, which totaled about five hundred yards, lasted no more than twenty minutes.

We emerged at the end buoyed by the shared family moment and the exhilaration of the cold. We rounded it all off with a hot chocolate topped with "whipped cream" and marshmallows.

I am intensely curious. One of my main drivers is curiosity. I want to understand as much as I can about life, the universe, and everything. But sometimes I realize it's more important to stop asking why for a minute and just accept that something simply is.

The magic of cold water is one of these instances.

Stepping into cold water, we intuitively feel its power, a growing sense of wonder and respect that is reinforced by our individual experience in it. We can encourage others to share the experience to see if it affects them in the same way.

Water is soft but powerful, fluid and dynamic, flowing, still, reflective.

Being the gloriously contradictory, complex, multilayered beings that we are, we would do well to heed the advice of philosopher-turned-Kung-Fu action hero Bruce Lee, who gently reminded us to "be water, my friend."

Perhaps we will begin to understand what is happening through a process that flows, like water, into the gaps in our knowledge. Then again, like magic, it may never be possible to understand the interrelation of physics, physiology, and neuroscience underlying our relationship with cold water. Yet we will still be able to feel soft, strong, and resilient as we go with and in the flow of the water.

Perhaps magical isn't quite the right word.

Alchemical, then.

Water has transformative powers.

We go in as one person and come out a better one. Base metal turned into gold. Reoriented, transformed, and more deeply connected.

For me, the quieting of my mind and the easing of my cares makes my cold water swim always worth the effort. I emerge from the water calmer and kinder. A colleague once described me as "very Zen." At the same time, my cold water swims also speed me up: At work, I sometimes become conscious of the fact that I'm on a more energetic level than everyone around me. Not because of a greater sense of urgency or a greater degree of stress, but thanks to the water's loosening of my limbs and mind. Because of that unconscious boost of energy, I move smoothly and rapidly around the operating theaters.

For the other swimmers I have profiled in this book, the activity has had a more profound effect. They are ordinary people who have had quite extraordinary experiences.

Candice went from literally having a hole in her head to becoming physiologically whole and balanced again.

Rob, who at the age of twenty was a physical wreck, is now officially an Ironman.

Solveig was once controlled by her condition but now has it under her control.

Kirsti transformed from SAD to happy, a reluctant couch potato to a celebrated Queen of the Ice.

Rachel, who was struggling and lacking confidence, has since become connected, to both people and nature, grounded and strong.

Sam wanted to take his own life but now helps others make the most of theirs.

Caroline, whose external transformation is more obvious, has moved from a psychological dead end to a place of passion and engagement.

Sarah has succeeded in giving up her pills and becoming the mother she always wanted to be.

Martin—stiff, aching, catastrophizing—is now at one with his body and enjoys the experience of exhilaration it gives him and the healthier perspective he once thought impossible.

Lonely in his pain, trapped by his mental health issues, Grant has rediscovered his lost tribe and become mobile again, and has more control of his pain.

David, who is otherwise trapped in his body and his chair, has found a window of relief, where he can move freely, without pain.

And Beth no longer suffers in stifling, darkened rooms. She learned how to escape from her disability and venture, at long last, into the bright and open, cold, clear water.

Further Reading and Resources

For occasional updates and interesting articles and videos about cold water swimming and lifestyle medicine, you can follow me on Twitter: @thecoldswimguy.

This section provides cold water swimming–related scientific articles, videos, websites, organizations, and books.

ARTICLES

Britton, Easkey, and Ronan Foley. "Sensing Water: Uncovering Health and Well-Being in the Sea and Surf." *Journal of Sport and Social Issues* 45, no. 1 (June 2020/February 2021): 60–87. https://doi.org/10.1177%2F0193723520928597.

Buijze, Geert A., Inger N. Sierevelt, Bas C. J. M. van der Heijden, Marcel G. Dijkgraaf, and Monique H. W. Frings-Dresen. "The Effect of Cold Showering on Health and Work: A Randomized Controlled Trial." *PloS ONE* 11, no. 9 (2016): e0161749-e.

Collier, Naomi, Heather Massey, Mitch Lomax, Mark Harper, and Michael Tipton. "Cold Water Swimming and Upper Respiratory Tract Infections." *Extreme Physiology & Medicine* 4 (2015): A36.

Cummings, I. "The Health and Wellbeing Benefits of Swimming Report." *Swim England* (2017). https://www.swimming.org/swimengland/health-and-wellbeing-benefits-of-swimming.

Denton, Hannah, and Kay Aranda. "The Wellbeing Benefits of Sea Swimming. Is It Time to Revisit the Sea Cure?" *Qualitative Research in Sport, Exercise and Health* 12, no. 5 (2020): 1–17.

Denton, Hannah, Charlie Dannreuther, and Kay Aranda. "Researching at Sea: Exploring the 'Swim-along' Interview Method." *Health & Place* 67 (January 2021): 102466.

Foley, Ronan. "Swimming as an Accretive Practice in Healthy Blue Space." *Emotion, Space, and Society* 22 (February 2017): 43–51.

Gundle, Leo, and Amelia Atkinson. "Pregnancy, Cold Water Swimming, and Cortisol: The Effect of Cold Water Swimming on Obstetric Outcomes." *Medical Hypotheses* 144 (November 2020): 109977.

Harper, Mark. "Extreme Preconditioning: Cold Adaptation through Sea Swimming as a Means to Improving Surgical Outcomes." *Medical Hypotheses* 78, no. 4 (April 2012): 516–19.

Li, Qing, Toshiaki Otsuka, Maiko Kobayashi, Yoko Wakayama, Hirofumi Inagaki, Masao Katusmata, Yukiyo Hirata et al. "Acute Effects of Walking in Forest Environments on Cardiovascular and Metabolic Parameters." *European Journal of Applied Physiology* 111, no. 11 (November 2011): 2845–53.

Massey, Heather, Ngianga Kandala, Candice Davis, Mark Harper, Paul Gorczynski, and Hannah Denton. "Mood and Well-Being of Novice Open Water Swimmers and Controls During an Introductory Outdoor Swimming Programme: A Feasibility Study." *Lifestyle Medicine* 1 (November 2020): e12.

Mole, Tom B., and Pieter Mackeith. "Cold Forced Open-Water Swimming: A Natural Intervention to Improve Postoperative Pain and

Mobilisation Outcomes?" *BMJ Case Reports* 2018 (2018).

Stephens, Richard, John Atkins, and Andrew Kingston. "Swearing as a Response to Pain." *Neuroreport* 20, no. 12 (August 2009): 1056–60.

Tipton, Michael. "The Initial Responses to Cold-Water Immersion in Man." *Clinical Science* 77, no. 6 (December 1989): 581–88.

Tipton, Michael, N. Collier, Heather Massey, Jo Corbett, and Mark Harper. "Cold Water Immersion: Kill or Cure?" *Experimental Physiology* 102 (August 2017): 1335–55. https://physoc.onlinelibrary.wiley.com/doi/abs/10.1113/EP086283.

van Tulleken, Christoffer, Michael Tipton, Heather Massey, and Mark Harper. "Open Water Swimming as a Treatment for Major Depressive Disorder." *BMJ Case Reports* 2018 (August 2018).

White, Mathew P., Lewis R. Elliott, Mireia Gascon, Bethany Roberts, and Lora E. Fleming. "Blue Space, Health and Well-Being: A Narrative Overview and Synthesis of Potential Benefits." *Environmental Research* 191 (December 2020): 110169.

VIDEOS

100 Days of Vitamin Sea, https://www.vitaminseafilm.com: This is Beth's wonderful film about her experiences of swimming with migraine.

Matt Baker, "The Countryfile Calendar Year," https://www.youtube.com/watch?v=-1rh-QLhMro: A profile of the Brighton Outdoor Swimming Club.

"Brave the Chill," ChillUK.org, https://www.youtube.com/watch?v=Rzk7gN6Ma68&app=desktop.

"The Cold Water Swim Cure—Ocean Therapy," Pechakucha, https://www.pechakucha.com/presentations/the-cold-water-swimming

-cure-ocean-therapy: This is a summary of the benefits of cold water swimming in twenty slides.

Fin and Jack Davies, "Hydrotherapy: Overcoming a Life Changing Illness through Wild Swimming," Friction Collective, https://www.youtube.com/watch?v=9Oe5Qnip9Bs: This beautifully shot film is about Laura Sanderson's cold water journey with fibromyalgia.

Mark Harper, "The Healing Madness of Sea Swimming," Head Talks, https://www.headtalks.com/healing-madness-sea-swimming-by-mark-harper.

"Sea Swimming Is 'Amazing' for Mental Health and Menopause," BBC, https://www.bbc.com/news/av/uk-england-devon-53851253: A BBC news report on the first Chill Therapy course.

"A Soothing Swim," BBC One, https://www.bbc.co.uk/programmes/p047z13f: This is a short clip featuring Sarah from Chris van Tulleken's program *The Doctor Who Gave up Drugs*.

WEBSITES AND ORGANIZATIONS

The Art of Manliness, https://www.artofmanliness.com: Although not a swimming website, provides lots of information about well-being and the outdoors; its podcast was a primary resource for this book.

The Bluetits Chill Swimmers, https://thebluetits.co/can-we-help.

The Breath Connection, https://thebreathconnection.org: Sam Murray's organization advocates conscious breathing, cold water therapy, and good nutrition.

Chill Therapy, https://chilluk.org.

Coney Island Polar Bear Club, https://polarbearclub.org/pb-site.

Mental Health Swims, https://www.mentalhealthswims.co.uk.

Mind, https://www.mind.org.uk: This UK mental health charity offers advice and support for mental health awareness.

National Institute of Mental Health, https://www.nimh.nih.gov: This US research organization provides information and resources for mental health.

Ocean Set, https://www.oceanset.co.uk: Yet another Brighton-based group providing sea swimming courses and instruction.

One Billion Happy, https://www.onebillionhappy.org: A website and podcast devoted to helping one billion people become happier.

Outdoor Swimmer, https://outdoorswimmer.com: This magazine is a good resource for all things outdoor swimming.

Outdoor Swimming Society, https://www.outdoorswimmingsociety.com: Brilliantly curated and presented website with answers to all your questions. They have information on safety, wild swimming groups, swimming while pregnant, and much, much more.

Pool2Pier, http://www.pool2pier.com: This Brighton-based organization was probably the first in England to run outdoor swimming courses.

SeaSure, http://www.seasure.org: This Brighton-based organization provides courses and information on sea swimming.

WeSwimWild, https://www.weswimwild.com: Laura Sanderson's organization seeks to protect wild waters from pollution.

BOOKS

Cox, Lynne, and Martha Kaplan. *Swimming to Antarctica: Tales of a*

Long-Distance Swimmer. New York: Harvest Books, Harcourt, 2004.

Deacon, Anna, and Vicky Allan. *Taking the Plunge: The Healing Power of Wild Swimming for Mind, Body and Soul*. Edinburgh: Black and White Publishing, 2019.

Deakin, Roger. *Waterlog*. London: Vintage Books, 2000.

Dickson, Paul. *The Official Rules*. Mineola, NY: Dover Publications, 1979/2013: Nothing to do with swimming but a frequent source for concise nuggets of true wisdom—including Agnes Allen's rule.

Gooley, Tristan. *How to Read Water*. London: Sceptre, 2017.

Heminsley, Alexandra. *Leap In: A Woman, Some Waves, and the Will to Swim*. London: Windmill Books, 2018.

Kelly, Catherine. *Blue Spaces: How & Why Water Can Make You Feel Better*. London: Welbeck Publishing, 2021.

Laing, Olivia. *To the River: A Journey Beneath the Surface*. Edinburgh: Canongate Books, 2011.

Landreth, Jenny. *Swell: A Waterbiography*. London: Bloomsbury, 2017.

Minihane, Joe. *Floating: A Return to Waterlog*. London: Duckworth Books, 2017.

Nichols, Wallace J. *Blue Mind: The Surprising Science That Shows How Being Near, In, On, or Under Water Can Make You Happier, More Connected, and Better at What You Do*. New York: Little, Brown, and Company, 2014.

O'Mahony, Seamus. *Can Medicine Be Cured?: The Corruption of a Profession*. New York: Apollo Publishers, 2019: Not about swimming but a fascinating and balanced account of the way modern medicine is developing.

Parr, Susie. *The Story of Swimming*. Stockport, UK: Dewl Lewis Publishing, 2011: As far as I'm concerned, the definitive history of swimming.

Rew, Kate. *Wild Swim*. London: Guardian Books, 2008: A wonderfully written book with many fabulous places to swim.

Russell, Richard. "A Dissertation on the Use of Sea Water in the Diseases of the Glands: Particularly the Scurvy, Jaundice, King's-evil, Leprosy, and the Glandular Consumption." London: R. Owen, 1760.

———. "The Economy of Nature in Acute and Chronical Diseases of the Glands." London: John and James Rivington, James Fletcher, 1755.

Shapton, Leanne. *Swimming Studies*. New York: Blue Rider Press, 2012.

Sprawson, Charles. *Haunts of the Black Masseur*. New York: Random House, 1993: My favorite book on swimming; wonderfully evocative.

Starr, Rob. *From Starr to Starrfish*. Kibworth, UK: The Book Guild Publishing, 2013.

Start, Daniel. *Wild Swimming*. Freshford, UK: Wild Things Publishing, 2013: A guide to swim spots.

Taleb, Nassim Nicholas. A*ntifragile*. New York: Random House, 2012.

Thomson, William. *The Book of Tides*. London: Quercus Publishing, 2016: A beautifully illustrated deep dive into tides.

Tsui, Bonnie. *Why We Swim*. Chapel Hill, NC: Algonquin Books, 2020.

Acknowledgments

It's impossible to know where to start and, even more so, where to finish acknowledging all the people who have, in some way, contributed to this book. I have drawn on the expertise, experience, generosity, time, support, friendship, encouragement, hard work, shared water-based adventures, and evenings in the pub of too many people to mention. Although I will try and mention everybody, I will probably miss some anyway. For that, I apologize—even outdoor swimming cannot completely reverse the effects of aging on my middle-aged mind.

First of all, thanks to Mark Tauber, my publisher, for searching me out and giving me the opportunity to write this book. When I was a beach lifeguard, I used to work on my great novel in my head but never got further than half a sentence in the style of Anthony Powell. I think I am much more suited to writing a book about cold water swimming. Thanks, too, to Miles Doyle, whose editorial input has been absolutely vital in making the book readable. Our work together felt very much like a collaboration. Then along came Jeff Campbell, whose attention to detail and textual renderings took the book to the next level. Many thanks to Eva Avery, my publishing marvel, who dealt with so many of the details so capably and got the book onto the shelves. And to the rest of the team at Chronicle—Cecilia Santini, Beth Weber, Tera Killip, Brooke Johnson, and Michelle Triant: I have been humbled by everyone's hard work, belief, and support.

Reading Mike Tipton's research first gave me an inkling that cold water swimming could be used therapeutically. Subsequently, his input, encouragement, and support has brought us to where we are now. Not to mention his willingness to supervise my PhD so expertly.

Research is all about teamwork, and in this regard, I have been so grateful for the untiring contributions of many people, but particularly in setting up, running, and analyzing the North Devon and Portsmouth studies: Heather, Amy, Hannah, Naomi, and Naomi.

The key moment in all this was to actually get patients into the water in order to undertake a clinical trial using sea swimming as a treatment for anxiety and depression. In this regard, first and foremost, I have to thank Mike Morris for his skill, powers of persuasion, and persistence in bringing Chill Therapy to life, without which I doubt this moment would ever have happened. In less than a year, it has gone from nothing to taking more than two hundred people every week into the waves, safely and with amazing results. Not forgetting Chris van Tulleken, "The Doctor Who Gave Up Drugs," who brought Sarah's story to a national (and international, since the program is available in Norway) audience. But there are many other people who have worked hard to get to this point, including Bruce, Sam, James, Ashley, Caroline, and Active Devon.

I have also got to put a special mention in for Scott and David, my incredibly patient research "enablers," who have been with me since I began working in Brighton nearly two decades ago.

Then there is Brighton Swimming Club, which provided me with my gateway to the sea. I am constantly humbled by the time and energy the volunteers put in to keep it running: Jasper, who first suggested I try swimming in the sea; and Nigel, who has kept me fit enough to make the most of it.

Not to mention all the wonderful friends I've made through swimming. I am especially grateful to those who have spent many mornings and evenings expanding my horizons over strong coffee and fine ales: Malcom, Ali, Paul, Bob, Bob, Lindy, Batch, Mike (Counter), Sara, Mark, and my long-distance swimming partner, Nuala. And, of course, the providers of those lubricants: Harveys and Dark Star breweries, the Red Roaster, and My Coffee Story.

There is also the gang at SeaSure putting courses together for those who might not otherwise get a chance to swim in the sea: Charlotte, Sam, Fiona, and Charlie.

Absolutely central to the book are the extraordinary and open stories of the men and women who have borne their suffering lightly and with determination and resilience. It would have been nothing without them. My heartfelt thanks go out to the contributors whose stories make this book: David, Candice, Sarah, Kirsti,

Caroline, Grant, Rachel, Martin, Solveig, Rob, Beth, Andy, Dennis, Sam, and Sian.

I feel incredibly privileged to have had such friendly, supportive, hard-working, humorous, and skillful anesthetic colleagues—far too many to mention individually—in both Brighton and Kristiansand. It's also been an absolute pleasure to spend so much time with the anterior spine team of Mike, Mike (Colin), and Flo—not only in the operating theater but also sharing our mutual love of food, drink, and (BBC 6) music.

Last—and most of all—thank you to my family. The reason I've had the confidence to pursue a slightly unconventional path through life and work is because you have always given me such a strong sense of love and security. My family-family, Mum, Dad, Nick, and Adam; my extended family, Jane and Graham; and my own family, Renate, Erik, Oskar, Ib, Lego our dog, and Mildred and Louis, our cats.

Notes

11: *Russell wrote about a similar effect:* Richard Russell, *A Dissertation on the Use of Sea Water in the Diseases of the Glands: Particularly the Scurvy, Jaundice, King's-evil, Leprosy, and the Glandular Consumption* (London: R. Owen, 1760), 47, https://books.google.no/books?id=NSHa5u76G08C&printsec=frontcover&hl=no&source=gbs_ge_summary_r&cad=0#v=onepage&q&f=false.

12: *"On my worst days, I just wanted to sit":* Quotes by Sarah are from episodes one and two of Series 1, *The Doctor Who Gave Up Drugs* by Chris van Tulleken, BBC One, aired September 15, 2016, https://www.bbc.co.uk/programmes/b0b4nxwt. The full episode is no longer available online, but view the clip "A Soothing Swim," https://www.bbc.co.uk/programmes/p047z13f.

24: *"To enter wild water"*: Robert Macfarlane, "Patron Statement," Outdoor Swimming Society, May 2008, https://www.outdoorswimmingsociety.com/patron-statement.

25: *"all sorts of ammonia"*: Adam Nicolson, *The Sea Is Not Made of Water: Life Between the Tides* (London: William Collins, 2021).

31: *"emotions and feelings of anxiety"*: Easkey Britton and Ronan Foley, "Sensing Water: Uncovering Health and Well-Being in the Sea and Surf," *Journal of Sport and Social Issues* 45, no. 1 (June 2020/February 2021): 60–87, https://doi.org/10.1177%2F0193723520928597.

39: *"A measure of the degree"*: Mathew P. White et al., "Associations Between Green/Blue Spaces and Mental Health across 18 Countries," *Scientific Reports* 11, no. 8903 (April 2021): 1–12, https://doi.org/10.1038/s41598-021-87675-0.

39: *In 2019,* Psychology Today *published*: Linda Wasmer Andrews, "Can 'Blue Space' Provide Therapeutic Benefits?," *Psychology Today,* March 22, 2019, https://www.psychologytoday.com/us/blog/minding-the-body/201903/can-blue-space-provide-therapeutic-benefits.

40: *A different review of thirty-five*: Wasmer, "Can 'Blue Space' Provide."

48: *This phenomenon has been demonstrated*: Mark Stevens et al., "Better Together: How Group-Based Physical Activity Protects Against Depression," *Social Science & Medicine* 286 (October 2021), https://doi.org/10.1016/j.socscimed.2021.114337.

49: *"It means a morning meditation"*: Quotes by Mary Cane, Mary Powell, Sarah Saunders, and Hilary Townley are from "Winter Nymphs 2016 Kenwood Ladies Pond," Hampstead Heath, "Swimming Ponds," April 2016, https://www.hampsteadheath.net/swimming-ponds.

49: *In 2018, more than 7.8 million Englanders*: Swim England, "Key Swimming Statistics and Findings," November 2020, https://www.swimming.org/swimengland/key-swimming-statistics.

50: *A meta-analysis of 148 studies*: Julianne Holt-Lunstad, Timothy B. Smith, and J. Bradley Layton, "Social Relationships and Mortality Risk: A Meta-Analytic Review," *PLOS Medicine* 7, no. 7 (July 2010): e1000316, https://doi.org/10.1371/journal.pmed.1000316.

51: *"We embrace outdoor swimming's"*: Macfarlane, "Patron Statement."

52: *"Let's be clear," Macfarlane writes*: Macfarlane, "Patron Statement."

52: *"During the pandemic, it was"*: Julie Bosman, "This Is the Story of a Man Who Jumped into Lake Michigan Every Day for Nearly a Year," *New York Times*, June 11, 2021, https://www.nytimes.com/2021/06/11/us/lake-michigan-coronavirus.html.

62: *"The blubbery arms of the soft life"*: Ian Fleming, *From Russia with Love* (Las Vegas: Thomas & Mercer, 2012).

62: *"Existing randomized trial evidence"*: Huseyin Naci and John P. A. Ioannidis, "Comparative Effectiveness of Exercise and Drug Interventions on Mortality Outcomes: Metaepidemiological Study," *British Journal of Sports Medicine* 49, no. 21 (November 2015):1414–22, https://doi.org/10.1136/bjsports-2015-f5577rep.

65: *In 2018, heart disease was the leading cause*: Details in this section are from Salim S. Virani et al., "Heart Disease and Stroke Statistics—2020 Update: A Report from the American Heart Association," *Circulation* 141, no. 9 (March 3, 2020): e139-e596, https://doi.org/10.1161/CIR.0000000000000757.

71: *"cold water immersion is certainly not"*: Diego Peretti et al., "RBM3 Mediates Structural Plasticity and Protective Effects of Cooling in Neurodegeneration," *Nature* 518 (January 2015): 236–39, https://doi.org/10.1038/nature14142.

73: *"Panting with the exertion, he went"*: Fleming, *From Russia with Love.*

73–74: *A paper by Jonathan Stone and his*: Jonathan Stone et al., "Acquired Resilience: An Evolved System of Tissue Protection in Mammals," *Dose Response* 16, no. 4 (December 2018), https://doi.org/10.1177/1559325818803428.

75: *A recent study, published in* Experimental: Mohadeseh Gilak-Dalasm, Maghsoud Peeri, and Mohammad Ali Azarbayjani, "Swimming Exercise Decreases Depression-like Behaviour and Inflammatory Cytokines in a Mouse Model of Type 2 Diabetes," *Experimental Physiology* 106, no. 9 (September 2021), https://doi.org/10.1113/EP089501.

77: *"If people with depression show classic"*: Caroline Williams, "Is Depression a Kind of Allergic Reaction," *The Guardian*, January 4, 2015, https://www.theguardian.com/lifeandstyle/2015/jan/04/depression-allergic-reaction-inflammation-immune-system.

96: *"Almost anything is easier to get"*: Paul Dickson, *The Official Rules* (Mineola, NY: Dover Publications, 1979/2013), 5.

105: *One such study showed that swearing*: Richard Stephens, John Atkins, and Andrew Kingston, "Swearing as a Response to Pain," *NeuroReport* 20, no. 12 (2009): 1056–60, https://doi.org/1097/WNR.0b013e32832e64b1.

127: *In 2017, the US National Bureau of Economic*: David G. Blanchflower and Andrew Oswald, "Unhappiness and Pain in Modern America: A Review Essay, and Further Evidence, on Carol Graham's Happiness for All?" *Journal of Economic Literature* 57, no. 2 (November 2017): 385–402, https://doi.org/10.3386/w24087.

128: *"a socially dysfunctional relationship"*: Margee Kerr and Linda Rodriguez McRobbie, *Ouch! Why Pain Hurts, And Why It Doesn't Have To* (London, Bloomsbury, 2021).

129: *Nearly forty years ago, Harvard psychiatrist*: Arthur J. Barsky, "The Paradox of Health," *New England Journal of Medicine* 318 (February 1988): 414–18, https://doi.org/10.1056/NEJM198802183180705.

129: *"Depressed people," he argues, "are"*: Elisabet Kvarnstrom, "Depression and Opioid Use: Recognizing the Need for Dual Diagnosis Treatment," Alta Mira Recovery Programs, July 2017, https://www.altamirarecovery.com/blog/depression-opioid-use-recognizing-need-dual-diagnosis-treatment.

130: *One showed that, following dental surgery*: Y Nagao, et al., "Effect of the Color of Analgesics on Therapeutic Results," *Shikwa Gakuho* (April 1968): 139–142.

130: *Another study, which looked at the efficacy*: E. C. Huskisson, "Simple Analgesics for Arthritis," *The British Medical Journal* 4, no. 5938 (October 1974): 196–200.

130: *Indeed, a 2013 study found that when*: Marjolein Hanssen, et al., "Optimism Lowers Pain: Evidence of the Causal Status and Underlying Mechanisms," *Pain* 154, no. 1 (January 2013): 53–58.

132: *"A review of pain in"*: David Ayers, Patricia Franklin, and David Ring, "The Role of Emotional Health in Functional Outcomes after Orthopaedic Surgery: Extending the Biopsychosocial Model to Orthopaedics," *Journal of Bone and Joint Surgery* 95, no. 21 (November 6, 2013): e165, https://doi.org/10.2106/JBJS.L.00799.

145: *This is an opening scene from the 2020 documentary*: Most of the quotes by Beth are from the film *100 Days of Vitamin Sea* (https://www.vitaminseafilm.com), though some are from an unpublished paper written by the author.

146: *migraines rank alongside psychosis and dementia*: World Health Organization, "Global Health Estimates: Life Expectancy and Leading Cause of Death and Disability," 2020, https://www.who.int/data/gho/data/themes/mortality-and-global-health-estimates.

150: *In 2009, Professor Michael Depledge*: Michael H. Depledge and William J. Bird, "The Blue Gym: Health and Wellbeing from Our Coasts," *Marine Pollution Bulletin* 58, no. 7 (July 2009): 947–48, https://doi.org/10.1016/j.marpolbul.2009.04.019.

151: *"He seemed to see something shining"*: G. E. R. Lloyd, ed., *Hippocratic Writings* (New York: Penguin, 1950/1978).

151: *"a rolling blackout, a chain reaction"*: Andrea Elysse Messer, "Your Brain with a Migraine: Effect of Electric Currents," *Science News*. June 2018, https://www.sciencedaily.com/releases/2018/06/180627160334.htm.

152: *Researchers have discovered that the release*: P. J. Goadsby, L. Edvinsson, and R. Ekman, "Vasoactive Peptide Release in the Extracerebral Circulation of Humans During Migraine Headache," *Annals of Neurology*

28, no. 2 (August 1990), https://doi.org/10.1002/ana.410280213; and P. J. Goadsby et al., "A Controlled Trial of Erenumab for Episodic Migraine," *New England Journal of Medicine* 377 (November 30, 2017), https://doi.org/10.1056/NEJMoa1705848.

154: *In 2021, the incredible work of*: See the Lundbeck Foundation, https://lundbeckfonden.com/en/the-brain-prize.

160: *"Many people with fibromyalgia have"*: Mark Pellegrino, "Dr. Pellegrino's Advice for Exercising with FM, Fibromyalgia Action UK, May 13, 2018, https://www.fmauk.org/information-packs-mainmenu-58/booklet-mainmenu-135/28-general-information/information-booklet/228-dr-pellegrinos-advice-for-exercising-with-fm.

160: *In their study, scientists harvested the blood*: Andreas Goebel et al., "Passive Transfer of Fibromyalgia Symptoms from Patients to Mice," *Journal of Clinical Investigation* 131, no. 13 (July 2021): e144201, https://doi.org/10.1172/JCI144201.

163: *"For me, a flare-up starts"*: Nikki Marshall, "Fibromyalgia Flattens Me. Here's What Helps Me Cope with Constant Pain," *The Guardian*, June 30, 2021, https://www.theguardian.com/australia-news/commentisfree/2021/jun/30/fibromyalgia-flattens-me-heres-what-helps-me-cope-with-constant-pain.

170: *A recent review and meta-analysis published*: Brigida Barberio et al., "Prevalence of Symptoms of Anxiety and Depression in Patients with Inflammatory Bowel Disease: A Systematic Review and Meta-Analysis," *The Lancet* 6, no. 5 (March 2021): 359–70, https://doi.org/10.1016/S2468-1253(21)00014-5.

172: *This was at least better than the 1930s*: "Professor John Hermon-Taylor Obituary," *The Times* (London), November 18, 2021, https://www.thetimes.co.uk/article/professor-john-hermon-taylor-obituary-2kl7x6rpg.

184: *Around 5 to 20 percent of individuals receiving*: For more on PTSD and these figures, see "What Is Posttraumatic Stress Disorder," American Psychiatric Association, https://www.psychiatry.org/patients-families/ptsd/what-is-ptsd; "Post-Traumatic Stress Disorder," National Institute of Mental Health, https://www.nimh.nih.gov/health/statistics/post-traumatic-stress-disorder-ptsd; and "How Common Is PTSD in Adults?," National Center for PTSD, https://www.ptsd.va.gov/understand/common/common_adults.asp.

185: *"My heart was constantly racing"*: The anonymous quotes in this section are from "Post-Traumatic Stress Disorder (PTSD)," Mind, January 2021, https://www.mind.org.uk/information-support/types-of-mental-health-problems/post-traumatic-stress-disorder-ptsd-and-complex-ptsd/symptoms.

187: *These include the following five simple*: The advice in this list is based on Lawrence Robinson, Melinda Smith, and Jeanne Segal, "Emotional and Psychological Trauma," HelpGuide, February 2020, https://www.helpguide.org/articles/ptsd-trauma/coping-with-emotional-and-psychological-trauma.htm.

192: The information about and quotes by Jill Bolte Tayler come from three sources: Jill Bolte Taylor, *My Stroke of Insight* (New York: Penguin, 2008/2016); Jill Bolte Taylor, "My Stroke of Insight," TED, February 2008, www.ted.com/talks/jill_bolte_taylor_my_stroke_of_insight?language=en; and Jill Bolte Taylor, interview with Mo Gawdat, Slo Mo (podcast), May 29, 2021, https://www.mogawdat.com/podcast/episode/4ccadd7f/dr-jill-bolte-taylor-part-1-meet-the-four-characters-of-the-brain-that-run-your-life.

211: *Similarly, a study of Finnish winter swimmers*: Pirkko Huttunen, Leena Kokko, Virpi Ylijukuri, "Winter Swimming Improves General Well-Being," *International Journal of Circumpolar Health* 63, no. 2 (May 2004): 140-44, https://doi.org/10.3402/ijch.v63i2.17700.